Escaping the Narcissistic Abuse Prison:

Reclaim Your Freedom From Emotional Abuse, Gaslighting, and Toxic Relationships to Rebuild Your Self-Worth and Become Self-Empowered

By Joan Hannon

© **Copyright 2024 - All rights reserved.**

The content contained within this book may not be reproduced, duplicated or transmitted without direct written permission from the author or the publisher.

Under no circumstances will any blame or legal responsibility be held against the publisher, or author, for any damages, reparation, or monetary loss due to the information contained within this book, either directly or indirectly.

Legal Notice:

This book is copyright protected. It is only for personal use. You cannot amend, distribute, sell, use, quote or paraphrase any part, or the content within this book, without the consent of the author or publisher.

Disclaimer Notice:

Please note the information contained within this document is for educational and entertainment purposes only. All effort has been executed to present accurate, up to date, reliable, complete information. No warranties of any kind are declared or implied. Readers acknowledge that the author is not engaged in the rendering of legal, financial, medical or professional advice. The content within this book has been derived from various sources. Please consult a licensed professional before attempting any techniques outlined in this book.

By reading this document, the reader agrees that under no circumstances is the author responsible for any losses, direct or indirect, that are incurred as a result of the use of the information contained within this document, including, but not limited to, errors, omissions, or inaccuracies.

Table of Contents

TRIGGER WARNING 1

INTRODUCTION 3

CHAPTER 1: UNDERSTANDING NARCISSISTIC PERSONALITY DISORDER. 7
- 1.2 DECODING NARCISSISTIC TRAITS 7
- 1.3 THE PSYCHOLOGY BEHIND NARCISSISM 9
- 1.4 IDENTIFYING NARCISSISTIC BEHAVIOR IN RELATIONSHIPS 12
- 1.5 WARNING SIGNS AND RED FLAGS 14
- 1.6 GASLIGHTING AND ITS IMPACT ON REALITY 16
- 1.7 THE NARCISSISTIC ABUSE CYCLE 18
- SUMMARY OF CHAPTER 1 21
  - *Warning Signs and Red Flags of Narcissistic Personality Disorder* 21
  - *Abuse Cycle Awareness* 23

CHAPTER 2: THE EMOTIONAL IMPACT OF NARCISSISTIC ABUSE 25
- 2.2 EMOTIONAL MANIPULATION AND CONTROL 27
- 2.3 ISOLATION: BREAKING FREE FROM THE NARCISSIST'S GRIP 29
- 2.4 UNDERSTANDING NARCISSISTIC RAGE AND RETALIATION 32
- 2.5 CHRONIC STRESS AND ANXIETY 34
- CHAPTER 2 SUMMARY 35
  - *Emotional Impact on the Abused Individual* 35

CHAPTER 3: BREAKING FREE FROM TOXIC PATTERNS 37
- 3.2 CODEPENDENCY 37
  - *Interactive Exercise: Relationship Pattern Worksheet* 39
- 3.3 OVERCOMING THE FEAR OF CONFRONTATION 40
- 3.4 THE GREY ROCK METHOD: DEALING WITH NARCISSISTS 42
- 3.5 THE ART OF BOUNDARY SETTING 44
- 3.6 IMPLEMENTING THE NO-CONTACT RULE 47
- 3.7 NAVIGATING CO-PARENTING WITH A NARCISSISTIC EX 49
- SUMMARY OF CHAPTER 3 51
  - *Steps to Free Yourself From Toxic Patterns* 51

CHAPTER 4: REBUILDING SELF-WORTH AND CONFIDENCE 53

Reflection Exercise: Cultivating New Habits *55*
4.2 REDISCOVERING YOUR IDENTITY 55
4.3 OVERCOMING NEGATIVE SELF-TALK... 57
4.4 THE POWER OF AFFIRMATIONS AND POSITIVE REINFORCEMENT 59
4.5 EMBRACING VULNERABILITY AND GROWTH 61
4.6 THE ROLE OF FORGIVENESS IN PERSONAL LIBERATION 63
4.7 STRATEGIES FOR REBUILDING SELF-ESTEEM 65
4.8 CELEBRATING SMALL VICTORIES ON THE JOURNEY TO HEALING 67
SUMMARY OF CHAPTER 4 68
Steps for Rebuilding Self-worth and Confidence.................... 68

CHAPTER 5: PRACTICAL STRATEGIES FOR COPING AND HEALING....... 71

5.2 STAGES OF HEALING... 72
Reflection Exercise: Mapping Your Healing Journey..................... 73
5.3 EFFECTIVE COMMUNICATION TECHNIQUES................................. 74
5.4 CREATING A SUPPORTIVE ENVIRONMENT 76
5.5 JOURNALING FOR PERSONAL GROWTH AND CLARITY 78
SUMMARY OF CHAPTER 5 80
Strategies for Communicating Effectively *81*
Recommendations for Supporting Your Journey *82*

CHAPTER 6: A HOLISTIC APPROACH TO RECOVERY 86

6.2 EXPLORING VARIOUS THERAPEUTIC APPROACHES 87
Individual Therapy *87*
Group Therapy.. *89*
6.3 FINDING THE RIGHT THERAPIST OR COUNSELOR 90
Reflective Exercise: Exploring Therapy Options *91*
6.4 BUILDING A NEW, EMPOWERED IDENTITY 91
6.5 EMBRACING CHANGE AND GROWTH 93
6.6 MIND-BODY CONNECTION: HEALING THROUGH MOVEMENT..................... 95
Physical Activity *95*
6.7 NUTRITION AND SELF-CARE AS HEALING TOOLS........................... 98
Nutrition *98*
Self-care.. *100*
6.8 DAILY PRACTICES FOR EMOTIONAL RESILIENCE 102
Journaling *102*
Managing Stress.. *103*
6.9 MEDITATION AND MINDFULNESS PRACTICES 105
Gratitude *108*

    6.10 THE BENEFITS OF BEING ALONE 108
    SUMMARY OF CHAPTER 6 110
        Steps Toward Healing 110

CHAPTER 7: PERSONAL STORIES AND TESTIMONIALS 116

    7.2 LEARNING FROM OTHERS: CASE STUDIES IN RESILIENCE 118
    7.3 SHARED EXPERIENCES: COMMUNITY AND CONNECTION 120
    7.4 TRIUMPH OVER TRAUMA: PERSONAL NARRATIVES 122
    7.5 STORIES OF SURVIVAL AND STRENGTH 124
    7.6 EMPOWERMENT THROUGH OTHERS' JOURNEYS 127
        Reflection Exercise: Turning Obstacles Into Opportunities 129

CHAPTER 8: RESOURCES AND FURTHER READING 130

    8.2 ONLINE SUPPORT GROUPS AND COMMUNITIES 130
        Reflection Exercise: Finding Your Community 132
    8.3 WORKSHOPS AND SEMINARS FOR CONTINUED GROWTH 133
    8.4 RECOMMENDED BOOKS AND ARTICLES 135
    8.5 TOOLS FOR ONGOING SELF-IMPROVEMENT 137
    8.6 CRAFTING YOUR PERSONAL HEALING PLAN 139
    SUMMARY OF CHAPTER 8 141
        Resources for Your Journey 141

CONCLUSION 144

    SHARING YOUR JOURNEY TO FREEDOM 146

GLOSSARY 149

REFERENCES 155

Trigger Warning

Trigger warning: This novel includes content pertaining to the subject of narcissistic abuse, which could be upsetting to some readers. Readers who may be unsettled by this topic should proceed with caution.

Introduction

It was a sunny afternoon when Lisa found herself staring blankly at her reflection in the mirror, wondering where the vibrant, confident woman she once knew had gone. Her partner's voice echoed in her mind, a constant reminder of her supposed inadequacies. She had been caught in a cycle of blame, manipulation, and emotional turmoil for years—until this moment. The realization hit her with a force she couldn't ignore. This was not love; this was not what she deserved.

Stories like Lisa's are not uncommon. Many people find themselves entangled in relationships that erode their sense of self, leaving them questioning their worth and reality. This book is written for you, the reader who seeks to break free from the shadows and prison of narcissistic abuse. It aims to provide practical methods for rebuilding your life and helping you thrive again.

My inspiration for creating this book has to do with my own personal experiences and my observation of family and friends who have gone through this type of abuse. We have all had encounters with narcissistic individuals to some degree or another. It is my hope that this book will bring understanding and healing to you as you embark on your own journey and break free from the narcissistic prison.

The damage that a narcissistic person can inflict on another is beyond comprehension. It can feel like a nightmare that you will never wake up from. You can equate their abusive treatment as vampirish, where you have every bit of self-worth and self-respect sucked out of you.

There is hope in escaping this nightmare. Just as your freedom has been broken down systematically by the narcissistic abuser, your freedom can also be reclaimed systematically. As you add the essential tools you will need to escape from this prison, you will be able to break through all the invisible walls that have kept you confined. You didn't get into this prison overnight, and escaping from it will require a consistent, methodical, and well-thought-out plan using the maps and steps provided in the pages of this book. It will require chipping away at anything that stands in the way of freedom. This is a prison we allowed ourselves to be caught in as we were baited and lured in by the insidious personality of the narcissistic abuser. Their plans certainly work on us again and again, so our escape plan will require strategic implementation to overcome any obstacle we encounter. In the following chapters, we will break down every single blockage and hindrance that stands in our way!

The journey we will take together is one of empowerment. We will focus on regaining confidence, self-worth, and self-respect. You will find that you are not alone, and that healing is possible.

Narcissistic personality disorder (NPD) is a complex mental health condition characterized by an inflated sense of self-importance, a deep need for admiration, and a lack of empathy for others (Lidner Center of HOPE, 2014). People with NPD may exhibit behaviors such as manipulation, entitlement, and an inability to recognize the needs or feelings of others. Understanding these traits is crucial as we explore how they manifest in relationships.

Narcissistic relationships are more common than you might think. Due to their prevalence, a significant portion of the population may experience a relationship with someone exhibiting narcissistic traits at some point in their lives. The emotional impact of these relationships can be profound, leading to feelings of confusion, self-doubt, and isolation.

This book is structured to guide you through the transformative process of healing. We will start by examining the nature of narcissistic abuse, then move on to exploring ways to rebuild self-worth, create healthy boundaries, and break free from toxic patterns. You will learn how to recognize and overcome the effects of narcissistic abuse. This book will also provide exercises and reflections to facilitate self-awareness and personal growth. Each chapter is designed to offer insights and strategies that are both practical and actionable.

Before we begin our journey together, I want to take a moment to acknowledge your courage. Confronting the reality of narcissistic abuse is not easy. It takes strength to face the truth and a deep resilience to seek change. You are here because you have that strength within you. You can choose to stay in the prison of narcissistic abuse, or you can choose to break free. Breaking free will take commitment and work. Through the pages of this book, you are being handed all the tools you need to break down the walls and experience true freedom on the other side.

As you read through these pages, I hope to inspire hope and empower you to reclaim your life. Healing is a journey, and it is one that you do not have to undertake alone. Together, we will work towards a future where you can live with confidence and joy.

This book is more than just words on a page: It is a companion for your journey, a source of understanding and support. You have already taken the first step by choosing to read this book. Now, let's move forward together toward healing and empowerment. Change is not only possible; it is within your reach!

As shown by the illustration below, we always have pivotal choices that we can make on our life journey. We can choose to move to a free and more abundant life or continue down the same path we are presently on, where we will continue to experience a stagnant and less vibrant life. It is entirely up to us which path we choose!

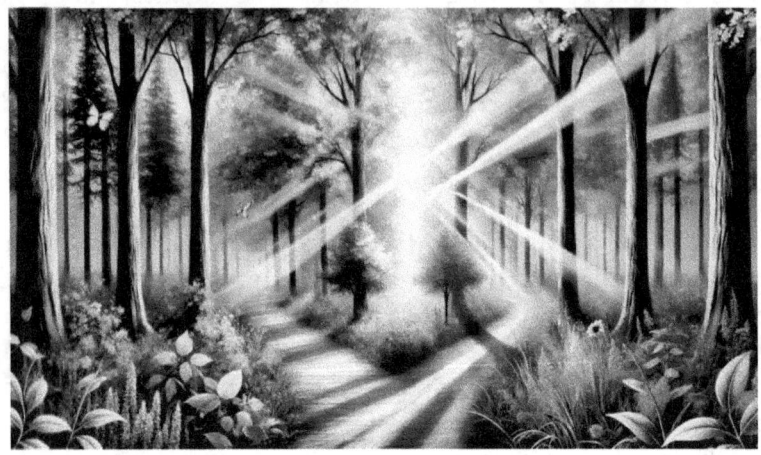

Chapter 1:

Understanding Narcissistic Personality Disorder

Have you ever felt like you were living in someone else's shadow, constantly trying to measure up to their ever-changing standards? It's a common experience for those who find themselves in relationships with individuals who exhibit narcissistic tendencies. These relationships can be overwhelming, leaving you feeling small and inadequate. In this chapter, we will explore what narcissistic personality disorder (NPD) really means, demystifying its traits and behaviors. Understanding these patterns is the first step toward reclaiming your sense of self and finding clarity in your experiences.

1.2 Decoding Narcissistic Traits

Narcissistic personality disorder is marked by a grandiose sense of self-importance, a need for excessive admiration, and a striking lack of empathy (Lidner Center of HOPE, 2014). These traits form the core of NPD, creating a complex persona that can be both captivating and destructive. Individuals with NPD often possess an inflated self-view, believing they are superior to others and deserving of special treatment. This grandiosity is not just about confidence; it's an unrealistic perception of one's abilities or worth.

Alongside this, there's a preoccupation with fantasies of unlimited success, power, or beauty. These individuals often imagine themselves at the pinnacle of achievement, even if reality suggests otherwise. They might believe they are destined for greatness, which can lead to frustration when the world does not conform to their expectations. This fixation on fantasy fuels their sense of entitlement and need for admiration, drawing others into their orbit with promises that seldom materialize.

Narcissism, however, exists on a spectrum. Some people may exhibit subclinical traits, where narcissistic tendencies are present but not pervasive enough to disrupt daily life significantly. In contrast, full-blown narcissistic personality disorder represents a more severe manifestation, significantly impacting personal and professional relationships. Subclinical narcissism might appear as someone who occasionally seeks validation, or has a high opinion of themselves, without the manipulative or harmful behaviors seen in NPD.

Covert narcissism introduces a subtler form, often characterized by introversion and hypersensitivity. Unlike their overt counterparts, who are bold and attention-seeking, covert narcissists may appear shy or self-effacing. However, beneath this exterior lies a hidden sense of superiority and entitlement. Covert narcissists might use passive aggression or play the victim to manipulate others, often leaving those around them confused and off-balance. Personally, I believe that covert narcissists are harder to recognize because of their subtle personality, which can make it more difficult to escape from that prison.

It's important to differentiate between healthy self-esteem and pathological narcissism. Healthy self-esteem involves a balanced, realistic self-view, allowing individuals to appreciate their strengths while acknowledging their weaknesses. This self-regard enables genuine connections with others and a willingness to accept feedback. In contrast, pathological narcissism is marked by an inability to see beyond one's inflated self-image, leading to defensiveness and a lack of accountability.

Understanding these distinctions can help you recognize when self-confidence shifts into narcissism, providing clarity in interactions that may have previously left you feeling bewildered. One example of healthy self-esteem might be someone who takes pride in their work and is open to constructive criticism. In contrast, a person exhibiting pathological narcissism might react with hostility to any perceived slight, unable to accept the idea that they are anything less than perfect.

As you reflect on these traits, consider how they might have manifested in your own experiences. Recognizing these patterns is crucial for making sense of past interactions and preparing for healthier relationships in the future. One way to start is by observing behaviors objectively, seeking patterns rather than isolated incidents. This understanding is about identifying others' behaviors and empowering yourself with knowledge and insight. You might ask yourself, *Is this a pattern that appears frequently, or is this a pattern that shows up infrequently?* Be vigilant with the feelings that you experience from the behavior patterns you witness and experience, but not over-vigilant to the point of obsession.

1.3 The Psychology Behind Narcissism

Understanding the roots of narcissism requires a look into the intricate web of factors that contribute to its development. Narcissistic personality disorder evolves from a combination of genetic, environmental, and cultural influences. Childhood experiences play a pivotal role in shaping personality, and parenting styles are often at the forefront of this discussion. Overindulgent parenting, where a child is excessively pampered or praised, can foster an inflated self-view. Conversely, neglectful or excessively critical parenting might lead a child to develop narcissistic defenses to protect themselves from perceived inadequacies. This dichotomy highlights the delicate balance parents must maintain in nurturing their children's healthy sense of self.

Genetic predispositions also contribute to the development of narcissism. While no specific gene is responsible for narcissistic personality disorder, research indicates that certain genetic factors may increase vulnerability to developing narcissistic traits. These predispositions, when combined with specific environmental triggers, can set the stage for narcissistic tendencies to emerge. It's akin to having a seed that requires the right conditions to sprout: Without understanding these genetic underpinnings, the full picture of narcissism's origins remains incomplete.

Modern psychological perspectives offer additional insights into how narcissistic behaviors are shaped. Social and cultural influences cannot be overlooked in today's world, where the glorification of self-promotion and individualism often prevails. The rise of social media platforms, for instance, provides fertile ground for narcissistic tendencies to flourish. The constant need for validation through likes and followers can exacerbate an individual's desire for admiration and attention. This societal shift towards self-centeredness can reinforce narcissistic behaviors, making it challenging to distinguish between healthy self-expression and pathological narcissism. I have observed individuals on social media platforms who appear to be obsessed with posting selfies, as well as posting their activities continuously. I believe it can become an addiction and a crutch that feeds on itself. The constant need for attention and validation through this venue can certainly breed narcissistic tendencies if that behavior is encouraged and allowed to persist.

More recently, researchers have delved deeper into the motivations behind narcissistic behavior to identify underlying insecurities and vulnerabilities that drive these actions. Despite outward appearances of confidence and superiority, many individuals with narcissistic tendencies harbor deep-seated fears of inadequacy. They construct grandiose facades to shield themselves from these fears, often at the expense of genuine connections with others. This understanding challenges the notion that narcissists are simply egotistical or self-absorbed; instead, it paints a more complex picture of individuals struggling with internal conflicts. Both the narcissist and the individual(s) they abuse are in a psychological prison.

The role of cultural norms and expectations plays a part in shaping narcissistic behaviors. Narcissistic traits may be inadvertently encouraged in cultures that prioritize achievement, success, and individual accomplishment. The pressure to excel and be recognized can drive individuals to adopt narcissistic behaviors as a means of coping with societal demands. This influence highlights the need for a nuanced approach when addressing narcissism, considering the broader cultural context in which these traits develop.

The intersection of these factors—childhood experiences, genetic predispositions, social influences, and cultural norms—creates a multifaceted backdrop against which narcissistic personality disorder can develop. Each element contributes to the complexity of narcissism, shaping how it manifests in individuals. Understanding these origins is crucial for those affected by narcissistic relationships, as it provides insight into the behaviors they encounter and offers a foundation for healing and growth.

As you reflect on these theories, consider how they might resonate with your experiences or the behaviors of those around you. Recognizing the psychological underpinnings of narcissism can offer clarity and empathy, fostering a greater understanding of the challenges faced by those with narcissistic tendencies and those impacted by them. In the end, exploring these origins sheds light on the disorder itself and illuminates pathways to empathy, growth, and change in the face of narcissistic dynamics.

1.4 Identifying Narcissistic Behavior in Relationships

Navigating a relationship with a narcissistic individual often feels like walking through a maze designed to confuse and ensnare. These relationships are marked by distinct dynamics, where power imbalances and emotional dependency become the norm. Narcissists wield control over their partners, friends, and colleagues by establishing themselves as the central figure in every interaction. They dictate the terms, leaving others to adjust and adapt, often at the expense of their own needs and desires. This dynamic creates a scenario where the narcissistic individual remains the focal point, while those around them are conditioned to orbit their whims and demands.

Key behaviors in these relationships often include manipulation, control, and a startling lack of accountability. Gaslighting, for example, is a favored tactic. This involves twisting reality to such an extent that the victim begins to doubt their own perceptions and sanity. It's a subtle, yet powerful form of emotional abuse that can leave lasting scars. Blame-shifting and denial are also common. The narcissist never accepts responsibility for their actions, always finding someone else to fault for their shortcomings or failures. Projection is another tool in their arsenal, where they attribute their undesirable traits or behaviors to others, absolving themselves of wrongdoing. These tactics, combined with smear campaigns and shaming, create an environment where the victim feels perpetually inadequate and anxious.

The cycle of idealization and devaluation is a hallmark of narcissistic relationships. Initially, the narcissist may shower their target with praise and affection, creating an illusion of a perfect relationship. This idealization can be intoxicating, drawing the victim deeper into the narcissist's web. However, this phase is often short-lived. Once the narcissist feels secure in their control, they begin to devalue their partner, subtly undermining their confidence and sense of self-worth. Criticism replaces compliments, and the victim is left questioning what went wrong. This cycle of lifting someone up only to tear them down serves to maintain control, keeping the victim off-balance and dependent on the narcissist for validation.

The psychological and emotional toll on those involved with narcissistic individuals is profound. Victims often experience intense feelings of insecurity and self-doubt. The constant manipulation and criticism erode their confidence, leading to anxiety and a pervasive sense of inadequacy. It's not uncommon for individuals in these relationships to develop symptoms of post-traumatic stress disorder (PTSD) as they grapple with ongoing emotional turmoil and instability. The environment created by the narcissist fosters a sense of dependency, where the victim feels trapped and unable to break free of the cycle, perpetuating their suffering even further.

For many, recognizing these patterns can be the first step toward healing. Understanding the dynamics at play in a narcissistic relationship allows one to begin reclaiming their sense of self. By identifying the behaviors that have kept them trapped, victims can start to see the situation more clearly and take steps to protect their emotional well-being. This awareness is not merely about labeling or blaming; it is about acknowledging the reality of the situation and empowering oneself to seek healthier, more balanced relationships in the future. Recognizing these dynamics can help one start making sense of the chaos, paving the way for recovery and returning to self-worth and emotional stability.

1.5 Warning Signs and Red Flags

In the early stages of a relationship, everything can feel like a whirlwind of romance and excitement. Sometimes, this rush overshadows subtle but significant warning signs. One of the most common red flags in relationships with narcissistic individuals is an overly charming demeanor. This charm can be intoxicating, drawing you in with flattery and attention that feels rare and special. However, beneath this charm often lies manipulation. Recognizing when this behavior becomes excessive or feels too good to be true is important. It can be a tactic to gain trust and establish control, making it crucial to remain grounded and observant.

Another key indicator is inconsistency in stories or exaggerations. Narcissists often weave tales that shift with each retelling, filled with grand claims or embellishments. These can be small details or larger-than-life narratives about their achievements or experiences. Take it seriously if you notice discrepancies between what they say and what they do. Inconsistencies may reveal a disconnect between their words and reality, hinting at more profound issues with honesty and self-perception. It might feel uncomfortable to question someone's truthfulness, but consistency is a cornerstone of trust. Without it, the foundation of any relationship is unstable.

Addressing these inconsistencies early in the relationship can save you enormous regret later.

Observing how someone interacts with others can also provide insights into their character. Watch for how they treat people they perceive as below them, or those from whom they have nothing to gain. Are they dismissive, rude, or indifferent? Do they change their behavior depending on who is watching? These behaviors can reveal a person's true nature, showing how they might eventually treat you. It's essential to look beyond how they act when they are on their best behavior to see how they handle everyday interactions and challenges. This broader perspective can unearth patterns that are otherwise easy to overlook.

Your intuition is a powerful tool when identifying narcissistic traits. If something feels off, trust that feeling. Intuition is your subconscious picking up on cues that your conscious mind might miss. That inner voice nudges you when something doesn't add up, or behavior doesn't match words. This isn't about paranoia or mistrust, but respecting your instincts. If you feel uneasy or notice persistent doubts, don't dismiss them. These feelings can guide you toward a more in-depth understanding of the person you're dealing with.

Becoming self-aware is another critical step in recognizing red flags. Reflect on your own experiences and interactions. Are there patterns of behavior that consistently leave you feeling uneasy or confused? Self-awareness helps you identify what feels right and what doesn't, allowing you to set boundaries before they are crossed. Consider maintaining a journal to track these observations and feelings over time. Writing things down can clarify situations that may feel murky and confusing. Over time, patterns may emerge, providing a clearer picture of the dynamics at play.

Seeing through the charm of the underlying behaviors can be challenging, especially when emotions are involved. But by paying attention to these warning signs and trusting your instincts, you equip yourself with the knowledge needed to protect your well-being. Remember, it's not about finding faults or being overly critical; it's about ensuring the relationships you cultivate are healthy and nurturing. Recognizing these red flags early can save you from heartache and guide you toward relationships that truly uplift and support you.

1.6 Gaslighting and Its Impact on Reality

Gaslighting is a term that many have heard, yet few fully understand until they find themselves ensnared by its insidious grip. At its core, gaslighting is a form of psychological manipulation used by narcissists to seed confusion and doubt in their targets. It involves a deliberate distortion of facts and a denial of reality, aiming to make the victim question their own perceptions and sanity. Imagine repeatedly hearing that your recollection of events is flawed, or that your emotional responses are irrational. Over time, this constant barrage can erode your confidence in your own mind. This tactic is not just about gaining power; it's about maintaining control over the narrative, ensuring that the narcissist's version of events is the one that prevails.

Several phrases and strategies are emblematic of gaslighting. Phrases like, "You're overreacting," "It's your imagination," or, "That never happened," are commonplace in the gaslighter's repertoire. These statements are designed to dismiss and invalidate your feelings, suggesting that your emotional reactions are excessive or unfounded. Another favorite is, "I never said that," a tactic that sows seeds of doubt about your memory and reliability. Imagine being told that the very words you remember hearing were never spoken. This can lead you to question your sanity and recollection, making it difficult to trust your own mind. Such tactics create a fog of confusion, where the victim is left doubting not only their interactions, but also their very sense of self.

The psychological effects of gaslighting are profound and damaging. Victims often experience a gradual erosion of trust in their own perceptions, leading to a distorted sense of reality. This manipulation can make you feel as though you're living in a perpetual state of confusion, unable to differentiate between truth and fiction. This constant questioning of reality can significantly impact mental health, fostering self-doubt and anxiety. You may find yourself second-guessing every thought and feeling, wondering if you are indeed overreacting or misremembering events. The constant undermining of your reality can leave you feeling isolated and trapped, unsure of who or what to believe.

Despite its powerful grip, there are ways to counteract gaslighting and reclaim your sense of reality. One effective strategy is to keep a detailed journal of events and conversations. By documenting occurrences as they happen, you create a tangible record that can serve as a reference point when your recollection is challenged. This journal becomes a valuable tool, helping you maintain clarity and counter the distortions presented by the gaslighter. Additionally, seeking validation from trusted sources—friends, family, or mental health professionals—can provide an external perspective that reaffirms your experiences. These trusted individuals can offer support and confirmation, helping you navigate through the fog of manipulation.

It is equally important to focus on actions rather than words. While the gaslighter may use language to confuse and control, their behavior often speaks louder than their words. Observing patterns and inconsistencies in actions can help you discern the truth. This approach requires a conscious effort to detach emotionally and view the situation objectively, a challenging but empowering step toward regaining control over your perceptions. You are not alone in this struggle, and recognizing the tactics of gaslighting is a crucial step in preserving your mental well-being and autonomy.

Recognizing and understanding gaslighting arms you with the knowledge needed to defend against it. This awareness empowers you to protect your reality and fosters resilience and self-trust. As you equip yourself with these strategies, you will be prepared to face manipulation with clarity and confidence. You have the power to reclaim your reality and trust in your perceptions, forging a path toward healing and self-empowerment.

1.7 The Narcissistic Abuse Cycle

The narcissistic abuse cycle is a bewildering pattern that countless individuals find themselves trapped in, often without even realizing it. At its core, the cycle comprises three distinct phases: idealization, devaluation, and discard. During the idealization phase, the narcissist showers their target with admiration and attention. This period, often referred to as "love bombing," is marked by grand gestures, excessive flattery, and an intensity that feels like a whirlwind romance. The narcissist presents themselves as the perfect partner, drawing their victim into a false sense of security and connection. It's a carefully crafted illusion designed to make the victim feel special and irreplaceable.

However, this idyllic phase is not meant to last. The devaluation phase creeps in subtly, often catching the victim off guard. Small criticisms replace compliments, and the once-adoring partner begins to find fault in everything the victim does. This stage can be incredibly confusing, as the narcissist's behavior shifts from loving to contemptuous seemingly overnight. In this phase, the victim begins to question themselves, wondering what they did to cause the change. The narcissist's tactics are insidious, employing passive-aggressive remarks and manipulative behaviors to erode the victim's self-esteem gradually. The aim is to keep the victim off-balance, unsure of their own worth, and desperate to reclaim the affection that once seemed so freely given.

Eventually, the relationship reaches the discard phase. Here, the narcissist abruptly ends the connection, often leaving the victim with little explanation or closure. This sudden withdrawal is devastating, as it comes after a prolonged period of emotional turmoil. The victim is left to grapple with feelings of rejection and abandonment, struggling to understand how they went from being cherished to being discarded. The narcissist may move on quickly, seeking a new source of admiration and leaving the former victim to pick up the pieces. This stage solidifies the cycle, as the victim often finds themselves drawn back into the narcissist's orbit, hoping to regain their previous status.

A key tactic employed by narcissists throughout this cycle is intermittent reinforcement. This psychological strategy involves providing random, unpredictable acts of kindness amidst the chaos. These acts serve to keep the victim hopeful, believing that the loving partner they once knew can be reclaimed. It's a powerful tool of control, creating a push-pull dynamic that leaves the victim emotionally tethered. Just when the victim is ready to walk away, the narcissist may offer a gesture of affection or a glimpse of the idealization phase, reigniting the victim's hope for change.

Consider the story of a woman who found herself in a relationship with a man who initially seemed perfect. He was attentive, showered her with gifts, and made her feel like the center of his universe. But over time, subtle criticisms crept in. He began to belittle her achievements, comparing her unfavorably to others. These comments were often followed by apologies and small acts of kindness, keeping her tethered to the relationship. Eventually, he left without warning, leaving her questioning her worth and wondering if she was to blame. This emotional rollercoaster took a toll on her mental health, leading to anxiety and a profound sense of loss.

The emotional impact of the narcissistic abuse cycle is profound and far-reaching. Victims often describe feeling as though they are on an emotional rollercoaster, their self-esteem rising and falling with each twist and turn. The cycle fosters dependency, as the victim clings to the hope of returning to the idealization phase. This dependency is further exacerbated by the narcissist's manipulation, which leaves the victim questioning their own reality and doubting their perceptions. The constant oscillation between affection and disdain can lead to severe emotional distress, including depression, anxiety, and even post-traumatic stress disorder (PTSD). This can be described as psychological warfare and torture against another human being who has done nothing to deserve this deplorable treatment.

Navigating this cycle requires an understanding of its mechanics and a recognition of its emotional toll. Awareness is the first step toward breaking free, empowering victims to reclaim their autonomy, and begin the process of healing. Acknowledging the cycle's existence allows victims to see through the narcissist's manipulations, fostering resilience and the courage to seek healthier, more balanced relationships in the future.

SUMMARY of CHAPTER 1

Warning Signs and Red Flags of Narcissistic Personality Disorder

- grandiose sense of self-importance
- need for excessive admiration
- striking lack of empathy
- inflated self-view, believing they are superior to others and deserve special treatment
- preoccupation with fantasies of unlimited success, power, or beauty
- unable to accept constructive criticism
- control
- manipulation
- gaslighting
- projection
- blame shifting and denial
- overly charming demeanor
- discrepancies between what they say and what they do

- inconsistencies in stories or exaggerations
- derogatory treatment of others
    - changing behavior depending on who is watching
- smear campaigns and shaming
- rage and retaliation

Diagram of the Narcissistic Abuse Cycle

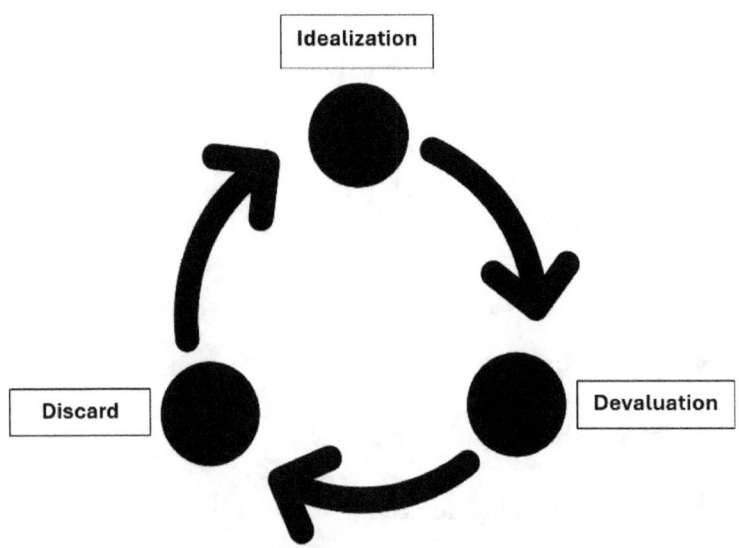

Abuse Cycle Awareness

- Recognize narcissistic personality disorder patterns.

- Trust your intuition.

- If something feels off, trust that feeling.

- Self-awareness helps you identify what feels right and what doesn't.

- Seek external perspectives from friends or mental health professionals.

Chapter 2:

The Emotional Impact of Narcissistic Abuse

Imagine a beautiful vase, crafted with care and precision, suddenly shattered into countless pieces. This is the emotional aftermath many experience after enduring narcissistic abuse. The once-whole sense of self, carefully built over the years, lies in fragments. Narcissistic abuse wields a powerful, undermining force, leaving in its wake a trail of self-doubt and confusion. You may find yourself questioning every decision and replaying scenarios in your mind, trying to understand where it all went wrong. It's not just about the choices you make now, but also the haunting echo of past decisions that never seems to leave your thoughts.

This chronic self-doubt is one of the most insidious effects of narcissistic abuse. It creeps in slowly, like a fog rolling over your mind, making you second-guess even the simplest of decisions. A constant stream of negative feedback from the abuser can lead you to internalize these criticisms, skewing your perception of reality. When you hear repeatedly that your feelings are irrational or your choices are flawed, you begin to believe it. This erosion of confidence doesn't happen overnight. It's a gradual process, chipping away at your trust in your own judgment until you feel paralyzed in the face of everyday choices.

Over time, this self-doubt can lead to a significant loss of identity. Living under the shadow of a narcissist often means adapting who you are to meet their expectations. You might find yourself changing hobbies or interests to align with theirs, or suppressing your true personality to avoid conflict. This adaptation is a survival mechanism, but it comes at the cost of losing touch with who you genuinely are. The person you once knew yourself to be becomes distant, almost like a stranger. As you strive to please the narcissist, your passions and interests fade into the background, leaving you feeling hollow and disconnected from your own life.

The struggle for self-acceptance in the aftermath of narcissistic abuse is daunting. Survivors often grapple with feelings of inadequacy, comparing themselves to an idealized version of who they were before the abuse. It's easy to feel unworthy, believing that your worth is tied to the perception of someone who never truly valued you. This battle is not just with the memories of the past, but also with the present reality of trying to rebuild a sense of self from the ground up. Accepting yourself, flaws and all, is a journey in itself, particularly when your sense of self-worth has been so deeply shaken.

Narcissists hurt themselves when they abuse their relationships. Our closest relationships play a huge and supportive role in how successful and fulfilled we can become as we grow together. When the narcissist tears their closest teammates down, they also tear themselves down, cutting off the avenues that will bring them the most joy and satisfaction in their lives. You might compare this to playing a team sport, where the most influential and strongest team member can either add extreme value to their teammates when collaborative, or become the biggest hindrance to the success of the team when that person believes they are the only one that counts. We don't win in this game of life by going it alone and destroying the lives of others along the way.

2.2 Emotional Manipulation and Control

Emotional manipulation at the hands of a narcissist can feel like being caught in a web, where each thread pulled tightens around your sense of agency and self-worth. Narcissists employ various tactics to maintain this control, subtly influencing your emotions and actions to suit their desires. One of the most insidious methods is emotional blackmail. This involves a deliberate play on your emotions to coerce you into compliance. For instance, a narcissist might threaten self-harm or withdrawal of affection if you don't conform to their wishes, making you feel obligated to acquiesce to avoid perceived harm or loss. This manipulation isn't always overt; it can manifest through subtle guilt trips or veiled threats, leaving you feeling trapped in a cycle of compliance.

Another common tactic is the narcissist's tendency to play the victim. This strategy allows them to avoid accountability for their actions by casting themselves as the wronged party. By portraying themselves as misunderstood or unfairly treated, they elicit sympathy and deflect criticism. This manipulation can make you feel responsible for their emotional state, pushing you to prioritize their needs over your own. In such scenarios, you might find yourself apologizing for things you haven't done or bending over backward to alleviate their supposed suffering. The narcissist's feigned vulnerability becomes a tool for control, keeping you enmeshed in their narrative and overshadowing your own needs and feelings.

Guilt and shame are powerful levers in the narcissist's toolkit. They exploit these emotions to deepen their hold on you, using your own conscience as a weapon. You might be made to feel responsible for their happiness or emotional stability, as if their moods are a direct reflection of your actions. This manipulation can lead to a pervasive sense of guilt, where you internalize blame for any negative outcome in the relationship. The narcissist's ability to shift responsibility onto you fosters a cycle of self-reproach and anxiety, making it difficult to assert your boundaries or express dissent. Over time, this can erode your sense of personal autonomy, leaving you feeling helpless and dependent on their approval.

The psychological impact of this control is profound and often leaves lasting scars. As the narcissist tightens their grip, you may begin to lose sight of your own autonomy, feeling as though you are merely an extension of their will. This dependency can manifest as a reluctance to make independent decisions or a constant need for validation. The fear of retribution or withdrawal of affection keeps you tethered, stifling your ability to act freely or voice your opinions. This loss of autonomy is not just about control; it's about stripping away your sense of self-determination, leaving you feeling trapped in a reality dictated by the narcissist's whims.

Recognizing these tactics is crucial to regaining control over your life. Awareness is your first line of defense against manipulation. By identifying patterns of emotional blackmail or victim-playing, you can begin to untangle yourself from the web of control. Setting clear personal boundaries is an effective strategy to resist manipulation. These boundaries define what behavior you will accept and what you will not, serving as a protective barrier against further encroachment. It's important to communicate these boundaries clearly and consistently, reinforcing them with actions rather than words alone. This might involve limiting contact with the narcissist, or refusing to engage in conversations that devolve into blame-shifting.

Seeking external perspectives can also be invaluable in resisting emotional manipulation. Trusted friends or mental health professionals can provide an objective view of the situation, helping you see the manipulation for what it is. These external voices can offer support and validation, grounding you in reality when the narcissist's tactics cloud your judgment. It's important to remember that you are not alone in this struggle; reaching out for help is a sign of strength, not weakness. By surrounding yourself with a supportive network, you can build the resilience needed to withstand the narcissist's attempts to dominate your emotions.

Breaking free from the grip of emotional manipulation is a process that requires patience and perseverance. It's about reclaiming your autonomy and rediscovering your voice, one step at a time. As you set boundaries and seek support, you will gradually regain the confidence to stand firm against manipulation.

2.3 Isolation: Breaking Free From the Narcissist's Grip

Imagine standing on a small island, surrounded by endless water, with no bridge in sight to connect you to the world beyond. This is what isolation looks like in a narcissistic relationship. Narcissists skillfully weave a web that cuts you off from friends, family, and anyone who might offer you support. They do this through subtle tactics, like expressing jealousy over your time spent with others or criticizing those you care about. Gradually, you find yourself making excuses to avoid social engagements, fearing the backlash of their disapproval. It's a slow process, often unnoticed until you realize just how alone you have become. The support network you once relied on feels distant, and the isolation deepens, allowing the narcissist greater control over your life.

The emotional impact of this isolation is profound. Loneliness becomes a constant companion, whispering reminders of abandonment and unworthiness. Without the comfort of trusted friends or family, you may start to question your own values, doubting whether anyone truly cares. This solitude can lead to a loss of social confidence, making the idea of reaching out seem daunting. The absence of external perspectives means you have only the narcissist's distorted reality to guide you, further entrenching their influence. You might feel trapped, as if the world has closed its doors on you, leaving you to navigate the tumultuous waters alone.

At its worst, a narcissist may draw you into a cult-like group that has isolated itself from society in order to maintain control and manipulation over its members. As they say, "There's safety in numbers!" This is a true statement. However, when used by narcissistic personalities, it provides them further insulation to maintain control over their own family, and to keep their family members isolated from the people who love and support them. I have personally experienced this insidious behavior, as a member of my own family was drawn into this web and trapped for 14 years. The detrimental effect it has on the family members inside the cult, as well as the family members who have been pushed away, is devastating. It takes many, many years for everyone involved to overcome this abuse. Don't be lured into the cult trap; it's much harder for you to reclaim your freedom once inside a group of this nature.

Rebuilding connections after such isolation is not just beneficial; it's vital for your recovery. It begins with small, deliberate steps. Reaching out to trusted friends, even if it's just a simple message or phone call, can start the process of re-establishing a support network. These are the people who knew you before the shadow of isolation fell, and they can help you remember who you are beyond the narcissist's influence. Sharing your experiences with them at your own pace can bring a sense of relief and validation. Remember, it's okay to lean on others. They want to be there for you, and your reaching out can be a healing process for them as well.

Joining community groups offers another avenue to reconnect with the world. These groups provide a space where you can meet new people and engage in shared interests, be it a book club, a fitness class, or a hobby group. Such activities can help rebuild social confidence, offering opportunities to interact with others in a non-threatening environment. Being part of a community reminds you that you are not alone, and it can reignite passions that may have been stifled by the isolation. It's about rediscovering joy in shared experiences and learning to trust the world again.

Community plays a crucial role in healing from narcissistic abuse. Engaging in group activities, whether in person or online, connects you with others who understand your journey. Participating in online forums, especially those dedicated to survivors of narcissistic abuse, can be particularly supportive. These forums offer a platform to share stories, seek advice, and find solace in the knowledge that others have walked a similar path. The anonymity of online interactions can be comforting, allowing you to express yourself freely without fear of judgment. Here, you'll find empathy and encouragement, helping to rebuild the social ties that isolation sought to sever.

The road to breaking free from isolation may seem daunting, but with each step, you will reclaim a piece of yourself that was lost. It's about opening doors you thought were closed and finding strength in the connections you've made. As you reach out and engage with the world, remember that you are not defined by the isolation you experienced. You have the power to rebuild, to reconnect, and to find a community that uplifts and supports you, no matter where you are in your recovery journey.

2.4 Understanding Narcissistic Rage and Retaliation

Narcissistic rage is an intense and sudden outburst of anger or aggression that can catch you off guard. It often occurs when the narcissist perceives a threat to their self-esteem or control. This perceived threat could be something as simple as a disagreement, or as significant as a challenge to their authority. The rage serves as a defense mechanism, a way to reassert dominance and quell any perceived insubordination. Imagine a volcano, dormant and seemingly peaceful, until pressure builds to the point of eruption. That's narcissistic rage—a volatile response to even the slightest challenge to their inflated self-view. Understanding these triggers can help you anticipate such outbursts, but it doesn't necessarily make them any less frightening.

When a narcissist's control is threatened, their reactions often escalate beyond mere anger. Retaliation becomes their weapon of choice, aimed at punishing those who dare to challenge their authority. One common tactic is the smear campaign. Here, the narcissist spreads false or exaggerated stories to damage your reputation. This can occur within social circles, at work, or even within the family, where the narcissist seeks to turn others against you. It's a calculated move designed to isolate and undermine your support network, making you more reliant on them. Financial manipulation is another tactic, especially potent if you share resources or depend on them financially. They might withhold money or sabotage your financial stability to maintain control, leaving you feeling trapped and powerless.

The impact of narcissistic rage can be devastating. Victims often find themselves walking on eggshells, fearing the next outburst and the consequences it might bring. This fear can lead to emotional withdrawal, where you retreat into yourself to avoid conflict. The constant anticipation of rage creates a high-stress environment, eroding your sense of safety and well-being. You might start to question your actions, wondering if you're to blame for provoking such fury. This internalization of blame is a common response, as the narcissist's rage often feels overwhelming and unwarranted.

To cope with narcissistic rage, it's crucial to develop strategies that protect your emotional and physical well-being. De-escalation techniques are valuable tools in managing confrontations, such as maintaining a calm demeanor, avoiding direct challenges, and using neutral language to defuse tension. It's about minimizing engagement without conceding control, and finding ways to steer the interaction away from conflict. Sometimes, however, the best strategy is to remove yourself from the situation entirely, if it feels safe to do so. Physical distance can provide emotional clarity and reduce the immediate threat of retaliation.

Legal protection options should also be considered, especially if the rage escalates to threats or violence. Understanding your legal rights and seeking restraining orders or other protective measures can offer a sense of security. Consulting with legal professionals can clarify your options and empower you to take necessary actions to protect yourself. It's important to recognize that seeking legal protection is not a sign of weakness; it's a proactive step towards ensuring your safety and establishing boundaries that the narcissist is forced to respect.

As you navigate these challenges, remember that you are not alone. The impact of narcissistic rage is profound, but it doesn't define you or your worth. You have the strength to protect yourself and seek a life free from fear and intimidation. In the face of rage and retaliation, your resilience is a testament to your courage, and every step you take toward safety and autonomy is a victory in itself.

2.5 Chronic Stress and Anxiety

The shadow of stress looms large in the life of anyone navigating the aftermath of narcissistic abuse. This stress is not just a passing cloud; it settles in, affecting both your mental and physical well-being. Imagine your body constantly being on high alert, as if an unseen threat is always on the horizon. This heightened state of awareness can lead to physiological changes like an increased heart rate, which feels like a drum beating persistently in your chest. It's also not unusual to experience sleep disturbances, where your mind refuses to quiet down, replaying past conversations and anticipating future conflicts. The impact on your physical health can be profound, manifesting as headaches, digestive issues, and even a weakened immune system. Over time, this chronic stress wears down your body's natural defenses, leaving you more susceptible to illness and fatigue.

The mental health implications of ongoing stress and anxiety are equally significant. Living under the constant pressure of narcissistic manipulation can exacerbate existing mental health conditions or give rise to new ones. Anxiety becomes a constant companion, whispering fears of inadequacy and failure. Depression can creep in, casting a shadow over moments that once sparked joy. For some, the stress of enduring narcissistic abuse can even lead to symptoms of post-traumatic stress disorder (PTSD), where the mind remains trapped in a loop of past trauma, unable to move forward. These mental health struggles can feel overwhelming, as though you're caught in a storm with no shelter in sight. The emotional toll is heavy, sapping your energy and motivation, making even simple tasks feel insurmountable.

In the face of chronic stress and anxiety, remember that reaching out for help is a sign of strength, not weakness. It takes courage to acknowledge your struggles and seek support. As you explore these coping mechanisms, be patient with yourself. Healing is not a linear process, and it's okay to have setbacks along the way. Celebrate the small victories and give yourself grace as you work towards peace and stability. You deserve to feel calm and confident, free from the constant grip of stress and anxiety.

CHAPTER 2 SUMMARY

Emotional Impact on the Abused Individual

- self-doubt

- loss of identity

- feeling inadequate

- feeling unworthy

- guilt and shame

- unmet needs

- loss of autonomy

- loneliness

- questioning your value

- walking on eggshells

- fear of retaliation

- chronic stress and anxiety
- mental health conditions
- codependency

Chapter 3:

Breaking Free From Toxic Patterns

Imagine sitting in your favorite coffee shop: The aroma of freshly ground beans is in the air and the comforting hum of quiet conversations surrounds you, yet your mind drifts back to a familiar argument from last night. It's the same argument you've had countless times before, with the same unresolved tension hanging between you and your partner. Recognizing these recurring toxic cycles is the first step toward breaking free from them. These patterns often manifest as cycles of conflict and reconciliation, where the initial spark of disagreement is quickly dampened by temporary resolutions that never address the root of the problem. You might find yourself emotionally dependent, relying on these brief moments of peace to sustain the relationship, despite knowing it is only a matter of time until the next argument.

3.2 Codependency

Emotional dependence can be a silent but potent contributor to these cycles. It's that feeling of needing someone else's validation to feel whole, to feel secure. This dependence often stems from a place of vulnerability, where your self-worth is tethered to another's opinion. You might notice that you constantly seek approval, bending your needs to fit the mold of what you believe will keep the peace. This dependence can blind you to the unhealthy nature of the relationship, as the fear of losing that validation overshadows the reality of the dysfunction. It's a delicate balance, where the comfort of familiarity often outweighs the discomfort of change.

Recognizing the signs of codependency is crucial in understanding these patterns. Codependency is more than just dependence; it's a deep-seated need to derive self-worth from the care and approval of others. You might find that you prioritize your partner's needs over your own, sacrificing personal desires to maintain harmony. This can manifest as a constant need for approval or an unwillingness to express your own needs for fear of conflict. You may even idealize your partner, overlooking their flaws and enabling their harmful behaviors. This dynamic can leave you feeling trapped in a cycle where your identity revolves around the relationship, rather than existing independently within it.

Reflecting on past experiences can shed light on how these patterns formed. Perhaps your childhood was marked by a need to please others, which was learned from observing parental relationships where self-sacrifice was the norm. These early experiences shape how you interact with others, often carrying forward into adult relationships. Understanding that these patterns are learned behaviors can be empowering, as it allows you to take control and make conscious changes. Recognizing the influence of your past enables you to address the root causes of your current behaviors, shifting the narrative from one of helplessness to one of empowerment.

Interactive Exercise: Relationship Pattern Worksheet

Take a moment to reflect on your relationships—past and present. Using a journal or piece of paper, create a worksheet that outlines recurring patterns you've noticed. Consider the following prompts to guide your reflection:

- What are common arguments or issues that arise repeatedly?

- How do you feel after these conflicts? Do these feelings linger?

- Identify any emotional dependencies—are you seeking approval or validation?

- Consider past relationships or family dynamics that might mirror these patterns.

Writing these reflections can help you visualize the patterns, serving as a starting point for change.

Evaluating your relationship behaviors through self-assessment can illuminate areas needing change. This involves looking at how you interact with your partner, friends, or family and identifying where these patterns arise. It's not about placing blame, but rather about understanding the dynamics at play. By acknowledging these patterns, you empower yourself to make informed decisions, paving the way for healthier relationships that prioritize mutual respect and individuality. As you embark on this process, remember that change begins with awareness, and each step you take is a step toward breaking free from the cycles that no longer serve you.

I know that keeping and maintaining peace at all costs is tempting, but this will only further erode your self-worth and self-respect. It will keep you ensnared in the trap of believing it's worth giving every bit of your independence away to please the narcissist. Remember, they will never be pleased with your codependency or any other self-preservation attempts. It only allows them to tighten their grip on you. Codependency can become a habit that will be hard to break as you seek to reclaim your life and your worth.

I have had my own battles with being a "people pleaser." If you can relate, then this personality trait may have started during your childhood, as mine did. It then becomes deeply ingrained later in life, to the point that it is difficult to deprogram yourself from this mindset. I have come to realize that it is not my job to attempt to please everyone else. Instead, I put my time and energy into becoming the best person that I can be, and I treat others the way I want to be treated. That is enough, and I am enough. Realize that you are also enough. You absolutely do not have to conform to what anyone else thinks you should be!

3.3 Overcoming the Fear of Confrontation

Confrontation can feel like standing on the edge of a cliff, peering into the unknown. The fear that grips you in these moments often stems from deep-seated anxieties about rejection or abandonment. It's a fear rooted in the belief that speaking up might sever ties, leaving you isolated and vulnerable. Many of us are taught from an early age that harmony is prized over conflict, leading to a reluctance to voice dissent. This fear can become a self-fulfilling prophecy, where avoiding confrontation allows toxic patterns to persist unchecked. The discomfort of confrontation looms large, often preventing you from addressing issues that need resolution.

Yet, addressing these issues head-on can transform relationships from fragile to firm. Healthy confrontation is not about conflict for conflict's sake; it's about fostering an environment where honesty thrives. By tackling problems directly, you open the door to mutual respect, where both parties feel heard and valued. This exchange strengthens bonds and encourages a culture of open communication. Imagine a space where you can express your feelings without fear of reprisal, and where your needs are recognized as valid. Such an environment nurtures growth, transforming relationships into havens of understanding and support.

Approaching confrontation calmly and constructively involves preparation and practice. Start by role-playing difficult conversations with a trusted friend or even alone. This exercise helps you anticipate potential reactions, allowing you to refine your responses. Preparing talking points in advance is another valuable tool. By organizing your thoughts, you ensure that your message remains clear and focused, avoiding the pitfalls of emotional overwhelm. Consider what you want to achieve from the conversation and focus on expressing your needs, rather than dwelling on past grievances. This shift in focus can help create a constructive dialogue that prioritizes resolution over recrimination.

Building confidence in self-advocacy requires practice in low-stakes scenarios. Think of situations in your daily life where you can assert your needs without significant risk. This might be as simple as expressing a preference for a restaurant, or voicing an opinion in a group discussion. Practicing assertiveness in these settings helps you develop the skills needed for more challenging confrontations. Remember, assertiveness is not aggression. It's about expressing your needs and desires respectfully and confidently, trusting that your voice deserves to be heard. As you grow comfortable in these smaller settings, you'll find that your confidence in more significant conversations strengthens.

The journey towards overcoming confrontation anxiety is as much about internal change as it is about external action. It involves challenging the internal narratives that equate confrontation with conflict and acceptance with silence. By reframing confrontation as a path to clarity and respect, you empower yourself to break free from the chains of fear. This shift in perspective transforms confrontation from a threat into an opportunity—a chance to assert your needs, strengthen your relationships, and reclaim your voice. As you practice these skills, remember that each step forward is a victory is a testament to your resilience and commitment to personal growth.

Baby steps will get you to where you want to go. It may be slow, but it's steady. In this case, you can be assertive without being aggressive or disrespectful. As the old saying goes, "You can catch more flies with honey than with vinegar." It is better to break down the walls of defensiveness than to cause the other person to fight back and defend themselves from an imagined danger. You can be honest and firm without being aggressive or pushy. This shows respect towards another and respect toward yourself. We don't always have to be right, or think our opinions are the only ones that count.

3.4 The Grey Rock Method: Dealing With Narcissists

Imagine being in a room filled with vibrant conversations and laughter echoing around you, yet feeling the need to blend into the background, unnoticed and unremarkable. This is the essence of the grey rock method, a strategy designed to minimize interactions with narcissists by becoming as uninteresting as possible (Fletcher, 2022). It involves providing short, non-engaging responses that strip away any emotional reward the narcissist might seek. When faced with a narcissist's probing questions or manipulative remarks, responses like, "I see," or, "That's interesting," offer little for them to latch onto. The technique encourages detachment, allowing you to maintain emotional distance and protect your well-being.

Knowing when and how to use the grey rock method is crucial. It is particularly effective in environments where cutting off contact isn't feasible, such as at work or during family gatherings. In the workplace, where professionalism must be maintained, employing this method helps avoid unnecessary drama or entanglement. When a colleague with narcissistic traits tries to draw you into office gossip or provoke a reaction, responding with minimal engagement keeps the interaction neutral and brief. Similarly, during family events where dynamics can be complex, this technique can shield you from getting entangled in old patterns. It's about creating a buffer, a protective layer that keeps you emotionally safe while fulfilling social obligations.

However, the grey rock method has its limitations. It's not a comprehensive solution to dealing with narcissistic behavior, nor is it effective in all scenarios. If you're in a situation where safety is a concern or the narcissistic behavior becomes abusive, this method may not suffice. It's important to recognize when more direct action, such as establishing firm boundaries or seeking outside help, is necessary. The grey rock method works best as a temporary measure to maintain peace without sacrificing your emotional health. It's about knowing when to use it as a tactical retreat rather than a permanent strategy.

The benefits of the grey rock method extend beyond immediate conflict resolution. By consistently employing this approach, you protect your emotional energy and reduce the likelihood of escalating confrontations. Narcissists thrive on emotional reactions, using them to fuel their sense of control and importance. By depriving them of this fuel, you effectively decrease their attention and influence over you. This reduction in engagement can lead to a more peaceful coexistence, where your emotional resources are preserved for more fulfilling and meaningful interactions. It's about reclaiming your emotional space, allowing you to focus on what truly matters without being drawn into unnecessary drama.

The narcissist is addicted to creating drama, so the less fuel you add to their fire, the better off you will be. Drama appears to be a drug that they can't get enough of, and as long as they can keep creating dramatic scenarios, they will get their "fix" until their next addictive craving. Anything you say that might threaten their power over you or keep them from their "drug" can and will be held against you. Give them no fuel by delivering passive responses, and the fire cannot continue to burn. Even if you have responses that make perfect sense, and they might benefit from them, they will never allow you to express yourself, as it is a threat to their control over you. Don't participate in their emotional and manipulative games. Seek out others in your support group that you can express yourself to and be shown the respect you deserve. This will build your self-confidence and self-worth.

3.5 The Art of Boundary Setting

Understanding the importance of boundaries is a cornerstone in cultivating healthy relationships and safeguarding personal well-being. Boundaries function like invisible shields, protecting your personal time and energy from being depleted by the demands of others. When you enforce boundaries, you create a safe space where your needs are respected, allowing you to nurture your identity without fear of encroachment. This protection is vital, as it prevents burnout and resentment, which are common pitfalls when boundaries are porous or nonexistent. Without these limits, you may find yourself constantly giving, yet still feeling empty and unappreciated—a cycle that ultimately drains your spirit. Establishing boundaries is not just about saying no to others, but also about saying yes to yourself, affirming your right to exist as an individual with unique needs and desires.

Defining personal boundaries requires introspection and clarity about what truly matters to you. Begin by identifying your own needs and limits, considering both physical and emotional aspects. Physical boundaries might involve personal space, privacy, or time management, whereas emotional boundaries relate to your feelings, thoughts, and beliefs. Recognizing your personal deal-breakers is also crucial, as they are the non-negotiables that protect your core values and well-being. Ask yourself what behaviors you find unacceptable, and what actions or words cross the line for you. This self-awareness empowers you to communicate your boundaries clearly and confidently, setting the stage for healthier interactions. It's about understanding what you need to feel safe and respected, and having the courage to articulate those needs without apology.

Challenges in boundary setting are common, but not insurmountable. One of the biggest hurdles is dealing with pushback or resistance from others. People who are accustomed to having unlimited access to your time and energy may react negatively when you begin to assert your boundaries. They might accuse you of being selfish or uncooperative, attempting to manipulate you back into compliance. It's important to remain steadfast, recognizing that their discomfort stems from a shift in the dynamic, not from your wrongdoing. Consistency in maintaining boundaries is another challenge. It can be tempting to relax your limits in the face of pressure or guilt, but doing so undermines your efforts and sends mixed signals. Stay firm in your resolve, reminding yourself of the reasons behind your boundaries and the peace they bring.

Communicating boundaries effectively is an art form that involves both assertiveness and respect. Using "I" statements is a powerful technique, allowing you to express your needs without placing blame. For example, saying, "I need some time alone to recharge," is more effective than, "You're always bothering me." This approach focuses on your experience rather than the other person's behavior, reducing defensiveness and fostering understanding. Setting consequences for boundary violations is equally important, as it reinforces the seriousness of your limits. Clearly outline what will happen if your boundaries are not respected, and follow through consistently. It might involve stepping back from a relationship, or limiting interactions until mutual respect is established. By articulating your boundaries assertively and respectfully, you lay the groundwork for healthier, more balanced relationships. Remember, boundaries are not about building walls, but rather about creating a safe space where mutual respect and understanding can thrive.

By standing firm, you can take back the territory you have lost previously by having your boundaries invaded time and again. Establishing and maintaining your boundaries will probably not be easy, as the narcissist doesn't like it when the rules of engagement are changed. However, you will be much happier and more fulfilled when you are consistent and unmoving in this endeavor. It's not showing disrespect to them at all; it is regaining your sense of self-worth and self-respect. Like anything, it will take work as well as resolve, but is invaluable.

3.6 Implementing the No-contact Rule

The no-contact rule is a crucial step in the healing process from toxic relationships, offering a sanctuary from the emotional chaos that often accompanies these bonds. At its core, the no-contact rule involves the complete cessation of communication with the person who has caused harm, creating a safe space where you can begin to heal and rebuild your life. This means no phone calls, texts, emails, or interaction on social media. It's about removing the presence of the person from your daily life, allowing you to focus on yourself and your recovery. This break from communication is not about punishment or avoidance; it's about providing yourself with the distance needed to gain clarity and perspective. In this space, free from the influence of the toxic relationship, you can begin to rediscover who you are and what you need to move forward.

The psychological benefits of implementing the no-contact rule are profound. By cutting off communication, you reduce the emotional triggers that can keep you anchored in past hurt and confusion. Without the constant barrage of messages or the anxiety of expected encounters, you can begin to breathe more easily, finding peace in the absence of turmoil. This space allows you to gain perspective on the relationship, seeing it with clearer eyes. Freed from the emotional fog, you can assess the dynamics more objectively, understanding what was damaging and why it thrived. This clarity is vital for personal growth, as it helps you recognize patterns and make informed decisions about future relationships. It's a period of reflection and self-discovery where you can focus on healing and reclaiming your sense of self without the interference of the past.

However, maintaining no contact can present its own set of challenges. Mutual acquaintances may inadvertently bridge the gap, bringing news or updates that you'd rather avoid. It's important to communicate your need for space to those around you, asking them to respect your boundaries by not relaying information. This can be difficult, but it's a necessary step in ensuring that your healing remains uninterrupted. Another challenge is the natural urge to reach out, especially during moments of loneliness or doubt. These urges are normal and can be intense, fueled by memories of better times or the hope of reconciliation. Overcoming these impulses requires self-discipline and a reminder of the reasons for implementing no contact. Consider journaling about your feelings or reaching out to a trusted friend for support, as both can provide comfort and reinforce your commitment to healing.

To effectively implement the no-contact rule, a systematic approach can help ensure its success. Start by removing the person from your social media platforms, eliminating the temptation to check their profiles or engage with their content. This step helps prevent accidental interactions and reduces the emotional impact of seeing their updates. Next, block their phone numbers and emails, creating a barrier that prevents unwanted communication. This act of blocking is a declaration of self-preservation, a commitment to prioritizing your well-being over the remnants of a toxic connection. If you share mutual spaces, such as workplace environments or social groups, establish clear boundaries. Inform those around you of your decision, and if necessary, adjust your routines to minimize contact. It's about crafting a life where you feel safe and in control, free from the shadows of past toxicity.

Remember, the no-contact rule is a tool for healing, not a magic cure. It requires patience and perseverance, as the absence of contact can initially feel like an empty void. However, over time, this space will be filled with self-awareness, strength, and new beginnings. It's a path to self-discovery and empowerment where you can focus on what truly matters—your growth and happiness. Each day without contact is a step toward a future untethered from the past, where you can thrive in the light of newfound clarity and peace.

Certainly, no contact can be difficult if you have been in a relationship with the narcissist for a long time and/or have children together. No matter your situation, it's possible to achieve no contact with some planning, and the benefits for you will far outweigh all of the emotional conflict.

3.7 Navigating Co-parenting With a Narcissistic Ex

Co-parenting with a narcissistic ex is like navigating a turbulent sea, where each wave brings a new challenge. The journey is fraught with difficulties, as inconsistent parenting styles and manipulative tactics often come into play. One parent might strive to create a nurturing environment, emphasizing stability and routine, while the other may undermine these efforts with unpredictability and self-serving behaviors. The narcissistic ex might use the child as a pawn in a power game, employing tactics to create tension and discord. This manipulation can take many forms, from bad-mouthing the other parent to bending rules to appear as the "fun" parent. Such behavior strains the co-parenting relationship and confuses and distresses the child, who becomes caught in the crossfire.

Amidst this chaos, consistency becomes the anchor that keeps the child grounded. Maintaining steady rules and routines is crucial to provide a sense of security and predictability. Children thrive in environments where they know what to expect, and this stability fosters a sense of safety and trust. Establishing clear guidelines for bedtime, homework, and leisure activities can help create a structured environment, supporting the child's emotional and psychological well-being. Consistency is not just about rules; it's about reinforcing the child's sense of belonging and stability, even when external circumstances are tumultuous. By offering this stability, you help shield the child from the emotional turbulence of a narcissistic parent's tactics.

Effective co-parenting requires a strategic approach to managing dynamics while protecting your own emotional health. Establishing clear communication boundaries is essential. This might mean limiting communication to written forms like email or text, which provides a record of interactions and reduces the likelihood of confrontations. Clear communication ensures that discussions remain focused on the child's needs rather than being derailed by personal grievances. It's important to remain calm and composed, avoiding reactive or emotional exchanges that could be used against you. Consider setting regular check-ins to discuss the child's progress and needs, always prioritizing their well-being over personal conflicts. This approach not only safeguards your emotional energy, but also models respectful communication for the child.

Navigating the complexities of co-parenting with a narcissistic ex often requires external support. Legal guidance can be invaluable, particularly in ensuring that custody arrangements and parental responsibilities are clearly defined and upheld. Consulting with a family attorney can help clarify your rights and options, providing a framework for navigating disputes and protecting the child's interests. In addition to legal support, emotional support is crucial. Attending co-parenting workshops can offer practical strategies and insights from professionals and peers who understand the challenges you face. These workshops provide a sense of community, reminding you that you are not alone on this journey. They offer tools to manage stress and improve communication, enhancing your ability to co-parent effectively.

As you navigate these challenges, remember that your resilience and dedication significantly impact your child's well-being. Maintaining consistency, establishing clear boundaries, and seeking support provides a stable foundation for your child to grow and thrive. Each step you take toward effective co-parenting is a testament to your commitment to your child's happiness and security. The path may be difficult, but your efforts ensure that love and stability remain at the heart of your child's experience. As you continue this endeavor, know that your strength and determination will lead your family toward a brighter, more harmonious future.

If your child's welfare is the primary focus when it comes to co-parenting, everyone will benefit greatly. Most importantly, your child will benefit when their parents model behavior that is mature and responsible. This is a positive tool they can learn to use in their own relationships with friends and family as they mature.

SUMMARY of CHAPTER 3

Steps to Free Yourself From Toxic Patterns

- Identify codependency in your relationship. This comes from a deep-seated need to derive self-worth from the care and approval of others.

- Overcome the fear of confrontation. Assertiveness is not aggression. It's about expressing your needs and desires respectfully and confidently, trusting that your voice deserves to be heard. Reflecting on past experiences can shed light on how these patterns formed.

- Implement the gray rock method by offering responses like, "I see," or, "That's interesting," which can effectively defuse tension. These phrases convey acknowledgment without engagement, signaling that you're uninterested in further discussion.

- Communicate boundaries effectively. This is an art form that involves both assertiveness and respect. Articulate your boundaries assertively and respectfully without apology.

- Implement the no-contact rule. This involves the complete cessation of communication with the person who has caused harm, creating a safe space where you can begin to heal and rebuild your life.

- Plan co-parenting strategies using clear communication to ensure that discussions remain focused on the child's needs rather than being derailed by personal grievances.

Chapter 4:

Rebuilding Self-worth and Confidence

Picture this: You're standing in a garden at the end of winter, looking at barren branches and lifeless soil. Yet, beneath the surface, life stirs, waiting for the warmth of spring to coax it into bloom. Much like this garden, your self-worth and confidence hold the potential for renewal, even if battered by narcissistic influence. This chapter is about nurturing that potential and fostering growth that leads to a life free from the shadows of narcissism. It's about planting seeds of new habits and cultivating a supportive environment where you can truly flourish.

Just like that winter garden, the environment you immerse yourself in is crucial to your recovery and growth. You can choose to stay immersed in a lifeless landscape, or immerse yourself in a landscape filled with new life and growth. Surrounding yourself with positive, supportive individuals and communities can act as a safety net, catching you when you falter and lifting you when you soar. Joining interest-based groups can foster connections that are rooted in shared passions and mutual respect. Whether it's a book club, hiking group, or art class, engaging with others who share your interests provides a sense of belonging and purpose. These communities offer a space where you can express yourself freely, unburdened by the fear of judgment or manipulation.

They become a source of encouragement, celebrating your progress and supporting your journey.

Personal growth is an ongoing process, a journey that requires dedication and effort. Setting goals for personal development ensures that growth remains a priority in your life. Start by identifying areas where you wish to improve or explore, whether it's learning a new skill, adopting healthier habits, or deepening emotional awareness. Break these goals into manageable steps, celebrating each achievement along the way. This approach fosters a sense of accomplishment and builds confidence as you witness your progress. Remember to remain flexible, allowing your goals to evolve as you do. Growth is not a destination, but a continuous process of self-discovery and improvement.

Gratitude plays a pivotal role in maintaining a positive mindset, particularly during challenging times. Cultivating a gratitude practice can help shift focus from what you lack to what you have. Daily gratitude journaling, where you jot down things you are thankful for, can create a reservoir of positivity to draw from on tougher days. Sharing gratitude with others, whether through a simple thank you note or a conversation, extends this positivity outward, strengthening relationships and fostering community. Gratitude acts as a balm, soothing the rough edges of adversity and reminding you that even in the midst of struggle, there is beauty and goodness.

In recognizing your victories and cultivating gratitude, you create a foundation for continued growth and resilience. These practices are not just about the present moment, but also about building a mindset that supports your journey forward, paving the way for deeper healing and fulfillment. As you continue to embrace these small wins, remember that each one is a testament to your strength and determination—a beacon lighting the path to a future filled with hope and possibility.

Building a life free from narcissistic influence starts with creating new, healthy habits that support your journey. A daily gratitude practice is a powerful tool in this transformation. By acknowledging the positives in your life, you shift focus from negativity to appreciation, fostering a mindset that nurtures self-worth. Consider starting each day by jotting down three things you're grateful for, no matter how small they may seem. This practice trains your mind to seek out the good, gradually reshaping your perspective.

Reflection Exercise: Cultivating New Habits

Take a moment to reflect on the habits you wish to cultivate. Consider how they align with your values and contribute to your well-being. Write down a few habits you'd like to adopt, and the steps needed to integrate them into your daily routine. Reflect on the impact these changes might have on your life, and the ways they can support your journey towards self-worth and confidence. Remember, the seeds you plant today will shape the garden of your tomorrow.

4.2 Rediscovering Your Identity

Rediscovering your identity after leaving a narcissistic relationship can feel like waking up from a long, disorienting dream. For so long, your sense of self may have been overshadowed by someone else's narrative, leaving you feeling lost and unsure of who you truly are. The process of self-discovery is about peeling back these layers, slowly revealing the person beneath. Reflective journaling is a powerful tool in this exploration. By writing down your thoughts and emotions, you create a dialogue with yourself, as well as a way to process and understand your experiences. This practice allows you to identify personal values and beliefs that are separate from the influences of others. Reflect on what matters to you, what you stand for, and what brings you joy. These reflections are the building blocks of your renewed identity, guiding you toward a life that resonates with your authentic self.

As you embark on this path, consider revisiting passions and interests that may have been set aside. Perhaps you used to love painting, writing, or playing a musical instrument before the demands of a toxic relationship overshadowed those activities. Reconnecting with these hobbies can reignite a spark within, reminding you of who you were before the clouds rolled in. Childhood interests are especially telling, offering insights into your innate preferences and talents. They are often pure expressions of curiosity and joy, untainted by external expectations. Allow yourself the freedom to explore these passions once more without the pressure of perfection or the fear of judgment. The act of simply engaging in activities that bring you happiness can be profoundly healing, nurturing a sense of autonomy and self-worth.

Self-discovery is not a destination, but an ongoing exploration. It involves embracing new interests and passions as they emerge, allowing your identity to evolve naturally. This fluidity is a testament to your resilience and adaptability, qualities that have carried you through challenging times. As you explore new activities, you may find unexpected joys and talents, further enriching your sense of self. Engage in activities that challenge you and push you out of your comfort zone. Whether it's learning a new language, taking a dance class, or volunteering for a cause you care about, each experience adds depth and texture to your identity, broadening your horizons and enhancing your life.

To assess your strengths and weaknesses objectively, consider using personality assessments or conducting a strengths and weaknesses analysis. These tools provide valuable insights into your character and capabilities, offering a clearer picture of your unique traits. Understanding your strengths allows you to leverage them in pursuit of your goals, while recognizing your weaknesses provides opportunities for growth and improvement. This self-awareness is empowering, equipping you with the knowledge to navigate life with confidence and purpose. As you continue this exploration, remember that rediscovering your identity is a personal and evolving process, one that celebrates the unique and multifaceted person you are.

4.3 Overcoming Negative Self-talk

Have you ever caught yourself saying things in your mind that you wouldn't dream of saying to someone else? The language we use internally shapes our self-esteem and confidence in profound ways. Words carry immense power, capable of building us up or tearing us down. When you constantly tell yourself that you're *not good enough* or *always failing*, these phrases seep into your subconscious, influencing how you perceive yourself and your abilities. It's like planting seeds of doubt that grow into a forest of insecurity. Over time, this negative self-talk can become a habitual pattern, one that quietly undermines your self-worth without you even realizing it.

Recognizing patterns of negative self-talk is the first step toward change. Common thought patterns include overgeneralizations, where a single mistake becomes a sweeping statement about your abilities, or catastrophizing, where you expect the worst outcomes in every situation. These thoughts often have triggers—stressful situations, past criticisms, or even a simple mistake can set them off. By identifying these patterns and their triggers, you can begin to understand how deeply they affect your perception of self. Awareness is crucial; it allows you to catch these thoughts as they occur, giving you the opportunity to challenge and change them before they take root.

One effective method for addressing negative self-talk is cognitive restructuring, a technique used to challenge and reframe unhelpful thoughts. Thought-stopping, for example, involves consciously interrupting negative thoughts as they arise, replacing them with constructive alternatives. When you catch yourself thinking, *I can't do this*, pause and reframe it to, *This is challenging, but I can learn from it*. This shift in language not only changes the immediate impact of the thought, but also gradually trains your brain to adopt a more positive outlook. Replacing negativity with constructive alternatives involves consciously choosing words that empower rather than belittle, fostering a mindset that supports growth and resilience.

Practical exercises can help reinforce this new way of thinking. Creating a positive mantra list is a simple yet powerful tool. Start by writing down affirmations that resonate with you, such as, "I am capable," or, "I am worthy of love and respect." Place these mantras where you will see them regularly, such as on your mirror or in your planner, and recite them daily. This repetition helps solidify these affirmations in your mind, gradually replacing negative self-talk with empowering messages. Over time, these positive affirmations build a foundation of self-belief, encouraging you to approach each day with confidence and assurance.

Overcoming negative self-talk is a process that requires patience and persistence. It's about being kind to yourself, recognizing that everyone experiences self-doubt, and taking proactive steps to foster a healthier internal dialogue. As you practice these techniques, you'll find that your self-perception begins to shift, allowing you to embrace your capabilities and worth with renewed vigor and clarity. Through this transformation, you reclaim your narrative, replacing doubt with determination and self-criticism with self-compassion.

4.4 The Power of Affirmations and Positive Reinforcement

Affirmations are simple yet powerful statements that hold the potential to transform the way we see ourselves. When you repeat affirmations, you engage in a form of mental training, strengthening positive pathways in the brain while weakening negative ones. Over time, consistent affirmations can increase your self-esteem and confidence. By affirming positive beliefs, you begin to shift your mindset, replacing doubt and negativity with assurance and optimism. This change doesn't happen overnight, but with regular practice, affirmations can profoundly impact your self-perception, gradually fostering a healthier self-image.

Crafting affirmations that resonate personally is crucial for their effectiveness. Start by identifying your personal strengths—those qualities and abilities that make you unique. Think about what you value in yourself, whether it's your creativity, resilience, or kindness. Tailor your affirmations to address specific needs or goals, ensuring they reflect what you truly want to believe about yourself. For instance, if you're working on building confidence, an affirmation might be, "I confidently express my ideas and perspectives." Keep them positive, present tense, and specific, focusing on what you wish to cultivate within yourself. Personalized affirmations serve as daily reminders of your potential, encouraging growth and self-belief.

Positive reinforcement plays a significant role in reinforcing self-worth. It involves acknowledging and rewarding positive behaviors, creating a cycle of motivation and affirmation. Establishing a self-reward system can be a powerful tool in this process. Consider setting small, achievable goals and celebrating their attainment with rewards that bring you joy. Whether it's treating yourself to a favorite meal or enjoying a day off, these rewards affirm your progress and effort, reinforcing the belief that you are deserving of success and happiness. By consistently recognizing your achievements, you build a foundation of self-worth that encourages ongoing growth and fulfillment.

To get you started, here are some effective sample affirmations:

- "I am worthy of love and respect."

- "I embrace change and welcome new opportunities."

- "I trust in my ability to overcome challenges."

Incorporate these into your daily routine, perhaps by repeating them each morning or writing them in a journal. Repetition helps embed these positive beliefs into your subconscious, gradually transforming your self-perception. Remember, the power of affirmations lies not just in the words themselves, but also in the intention and belief you bring to them. As you engage with these affirmations, you open the door to a more confident, empowered version of yourself.

There are various subliminal affirmation techniques you can research to see if there is one that resonates with you. For instance, I have used subliminal affirmations that I created with the sound of my own voice for many years now. The changes such techniques can make in the way you view yourself and how you handle challenges are extremely beneficial. By using some of these techniques, you can reprogram your mind from one of self-reproach to one of self-respect.

4.5 Embracing Vulnerability and Growth

Think about the last time you allowed yourself to be truly open with someone. It might have been a moment where you shared a fear, a dream, or an emotion that felt raw. Being vulnerable is often misunderstood as a weakness, but in reality, it is a profound strength. By embracing vulnerability, you invite growth into your life. It is through being vulnerable that we build authentic relationships—connections that are enriched by honesty and trust. Picture telling a friend about a personal struggle and finding not judgment, but empathy and understanding. This act of openness strengthens the bond between you and enriches your own sense of self. Many individuals who have faced their fears of rejection head-on have found greater fulfillment and success by embracing their vulnerability. They have learned that vulnerability is not about exposure to harm, but about the courage to be seen as we truly are.

Yet, many of us are held back by fears and misconceptions surrounding vulnerability. There's a pervasive fear of judgment—a worry that showing our true selves will lead to criticism or rejection. This fear is often rooted in past experiences where openness may have been met with misunderstanding or ridicule. But vulnerability is not about baring your soul to everyone; it's about choosing carefully who you trust with your inner world. Misunderstandings about vulnerability can lead us to believe that it makes us weak or overly emotional. In truth, vulnerability is a powerful tool for personal growth. It allows us to express our authentic selves, and fosters an environment where others feel comfortable doing the same. By redefining vulnerability as a strength, we open ourselves up to deeper connections and greater personal insight.

Practicing vulnerability can start in small, everyday interactions. Start by sharing your thoughts and feelings openly with those you trust. This might involve expressing your opinion in a meeting, or telling a friend about something that's been on your mind. It doesn't have to be a grand gesture; even small steps can build confidence and openness. By practicing vulnerability in daily life, you cultivate an environment where authenticity thrives. This openness invites others to reciprocate, creating a cycle of trust and understanding. As you share more of yourself, you build resilience, learning that vulnerability is not something to fear, but to embrace as part of your growth.

The growth that stems from embracing vulnerability is transformative. By allowing yourself to be open, you increase empathy and connection with others. This empathy fosters stronger relationships, where mutual understanding and support become the foundation. You'll find that as you practice vulnerability, you also develop a more in-depth understanding of yourself. This self-awareness nurtures personal growth, allowing you to align your actions with your true values and desires. Embracing vulnerability enriches your life, leading to connections that are genuine and fulfilling. It is a journey of discovery, where each step taken in openness and honesty leads to a more profound sense of self and a richer, more connected life.

As you practice vulnerability in your daily life, the walls you have built around yourself for protection will start to crumble and fall. Your vulnerability will be respected and appreciated when you are surrounded by people who truly care about you. You will begin to choose relationships that are healthy and balanced.

4.6 The Role of Forgiveness in Personal Liberation

Forgiveness is a concept often misunderstood, especially when it comes to healing from past wounds. At its core, forgiveness is not about excusing or condoning harmful actions. Rather, it is about releasing the emotional hold those actions have over you. It is about freeing yourself from the bitterness and resentment that can weigh you down, allowing for emotional peace and freedom. When you forgive, you are not saying that what happened was okay or that you are willing to reconcile with the person who hurt you. Instead, you are choosing to let go of the anger and hurt that keep you tethered to the past. This distinction is crucial, as many people struggle with forgiveness, believing that it means forgetting or pretending the pain wasn't real. In truth, forgiving is a personal act of liberation—a way to reclaim your emotional well-being.

Common misconceptions can cloud the path to forgiveness, making it seem like a daunting or even undesirable goal. A prevalent myth is the idea that forgiveness requires reconciliation. This belief can deter people from forgiving because they fear it means re-establishing a relationship with someone who has caused them harm. However, forgiveness does not necessitate contact or reconciliation. It is an internal process, focused on your healing rather than on the other person. Another misconception is that forgiveness is a sign of weakness. In reality, it takes immense strength and courage to forgive. It involves confronting your pain, acknowledging it, and then choosing to move beyond it. By dispelling these myths, you open yourself to the true power and potential of forgiveness as a tool for personal liberation.

The benefits of forgiveness extend beyond emotional relief, influencing various aspects of your mental health as well. Letting go of resentment can significantly improve your psychological well-being. Holding on to anger and bitterness can lead to stress, anxiety, and even depression. By forgiving, you release these burdens, allowing for a more peaceful state of mind. The act of forgiveness can also lead to improved relationships—not only with others, but also with yourself. It fosters self-compassion, enabling you to treat yourself with kindness and understanding. As you let go of grudges, you make room for positive emotions and experiences, paving the way for a more fulfilling and balanced life.

Forgiving yourself and others is a process that can be approached methodically, with intention and care. One effective strategy is writing forgiveness letters. These letters are not necessarily meant to be sent; rather, they serve as a means of expressing your feelings and releasing them. Begin by writing a letter to the person who has hurt you, detailing the impact of their actions and how you felt. Allow yourself to express any anger, sadness, or disappointment. Then, when you're ready, write about your decision to forgive, focusing on the freedom and peace you seek. You might also consider writing a letter to yourself, offering forgiveness for any perceived mistakes or shortcomings. This exercise is a powerful way to articulate your emotions, helping you process and move past them.

Blame and unforgiveness can be non-ending. It is like a disease that will slowly but methodically break you down and affect your mental and physical health if you do not let your unforgiveness go.

Writing a letter to someone who has hurt you, but not sending it, will remove a huge burden of guilt and shame off your shoulders and allow you to heal. The act of confronting grievances by writing them down will bring a sense of peace and calm. Unforgiveness will no longer have a hold on you.

Forgiveness is a journey that challenges you to confront your pain and rise above it. It is an act of strength and bravery—a choice to focus on your healing and growth. Through forgiveness, you gain the power to transform your past into a source of wisdom and resilience.

4.7 Strategies for Rebuilding Self-esteem

Rebuilding self-esteem after enduring narcissistic abuse is akin to constructing a sturdy bridge over turbulent waters: It requires both patience and deliberate action. Some of these strategies for healing and rebuilding yourself are repeated throughout different sections of this book in order to emphasize their importance and potential impact on your healing when implemented. Repetition can and will reprogram your mind to think in ways that build you up rather than tear you down.

One of the most effective techniques for enhancing self-esteem is the practice of daily self-affirmations. You repeat these positive statements to yourself, reinforcing your worth and capabilities. Imagine beginning your day by standing in front of the mirror and affirming, "I am strong, I am capable, and I deserve love." Over time, these affirmations help to rewire your brain, replacing negative beliefs with positive truths. Similarly, positive visualization techniques can further bolster your self-image. Picture yourself achieving your goals, thriving in your relationships, and living a life filled with joy and purpose. This mental rehearsal boosts confidence and prepares you to face challenges with resilience and optimism. Any new creation begins with our imagination: We take a thought and build on it in order to produce something brand new.

A crucial component of enhancing self-esteem is cultivating self-compassion. Often, we are our harshest critics, particularly during setbacks. Practicing self-forgiveness is a powerful way to counter this tendency. It involves acknowledging your mistakes and offering yourself the same kindness you would extend to a dear friend. Instead of dwelling on past errors, celebrate your progress, no matter how small. Recognize that perfection is an unattainable ideal; growth lies in the learning process. When you focus on progress rather than perfection, you foster a nurturing environment for self-improvement. This shift in perspective encourages you to embrace your journey with grace and understanding, allowing self-esteem to flourish.

Incorporating self-care practices into your routine can significantly impact your self-esteem. Regular exercise routines, for instance, enhance physical health and boost mood and energy levels. Whether it's a brisk walk, a yoga session, or a dance class, physical activity releases endorphins, the body's natural mood elevators. Similarly, mindfulness practices, such as meditation or deep breathing exercises, offer a space for mental rejuvenation. They help quiet the mind, reduce stress, and increase self-awareness. By prioritizing self-care, you signal to yourself that your well-being matters, reinforcing a positive self-image. These practices serve as reminders of your intrinsic value and the importance of nurturing your body and mind.

Setting realistic goals is another pivotal strategy in rebuilding self-esteem. Achievable, incremental goals provide a framework for success, allowing you to measure progress and celebrate accomplishments. You can start by setting short-term goals. Perhaps it's reading a book every month, learning a new skill, or dedicating time each week to a hobby. Your confidence grows as you achieve these goals, paving the way for more ambitious long-term aspirations. Setting and achieving goals builds momentum, reinforcing your belief in your capabilities. It demonstrates that you are capable of growth and change, regardless of past experiences. Through these strategies, you rebuild self-esteem and create a foundation for a life marked by confidence and self-assuredness.

4.8 Celebrating Small Victories on the Journey to Healing

Imagine you've been climbing a steep hill, with each step requiring effort and resilience. Reaching the top, you look back and see how far you've come. Celebrating even the smallest victories in your healing process can provide a similar sense of achievement. These celebrations are not just indulgences; they have tangible psychological benefits. Recognizing progress boosts motivation and reinforces self-esteem, creating a positive feedback loop. Each acknowledgment of achievement, no matter how minor it might seem, tells your brain, *I am moving forward*. This positive reinforcement is crucial; it shifts focus from what remains to be done to what has already been accomplished, fueling further progress.

It's important to recognize each small step forward to truly appreciate your journey. Keeping a progress journal can be an invaluable tool in this process. Documenting your achievements, whether overcoming a fear or making it through a difficult day, serves as a reminder of your resilience and growth. Weekly reflection sessions can complement this practice, offering a dedicated time to look back, appreciate your efforts, and set intentions for the week ahead. These reflections are not about dwelling on what could have been better, but celebrating the progress you've made. They provide a structured way to acknowledge your journey, fostering a sense of accomplishment and hope.

Celebration doesn't have to be grand or costly to be meaningful. Creative ways to celebrate personal milestones include creating a victory board and visually mapping out your achievements and goals. This board is a tangible reminder of your progress, something you can look at whenever you need encouragement. Planning a self-reward day is another enjoyable way to honor your accomplishments. Whether it's taking a day off work to indulge in your favorite hobbies or treating yourself to a special meal, these rewards reinforce the notion that your hard work deserves recognition. They serve as a pause, a moment to breathe and appreciate the efforts you've made.

SUMMARY of CHAPTER 4

Steps for Rebuilding Self-worth and Confidence

- Surrounding yourself with positive, supportive individuals and communities can be a safety net.

- Setting goals for personal development can be started by identifying areas where you wish to improve or explore, whether it's learning a new skill, adopting healthier habits, or deepening emotional awareness.

- Rediscover your identity by journaling your thoughts and emotions:
    - A reflective journaling practice allows you to identify personal values and beliefs that are separate from the influences of others.

- Revisit passions and interests that may have been set aside.

- A personality assessment is used to conduct a strengths and weaknesses analysis.

- Address negative self-talk:

    - Use a cognitive restructuring technique to challenge and reframe unhelpful thoughts.

    - Create positive mantras by writing down affirmations that resonate with you, such as, "I am capable," or, "I am worthy of love and respect".

    - Cultivate self-compassion by practicing self-forgiveness.

- Practice daily self-affirmations. Repeat these positive statements to yourself, reinforcing your worth and capabilities.

- Practice vulnerability by openly sharing your thoughts and feelings with those you trust.

- Forgiveness is not about excusing or condoning harmful actions. Instead, it is about releasing the emotional hold those actions have over you.

    - Cultivate self-compassion by forgiving yourself for past mistakes. Instead of dwelling on past errors, celebrate your progress, no matter how small.

- Incorporate self-care into your daily routine:

    o Physical activity releases endorphins, the body's natural mood elevators.

    o Meditation quiets the mind.

- Set realistic goals to provide a framework for success, allowing you to measure progress and celebrate accomplishments.

- Keep a progress journal to document your achievements.

- Keep a gratitude journal to document all that you are grateful for.

Chapter 5:

Practical Strategies for Coping and Healing

Imagine walking through a dense forest—each step uncertain, the path obscured by shadows. This is how the journey of emotional recovery from narcissistic abuse can feel—complex, winding, and often overwhelming. Yet, just as a forest eventually opens into a clearing, this path also leads to moments of clarity and light. The road to healing is not straightforward. It's a multifaceted process that brings its own set of challenges and rewards. As you navigate this path, you may encounter emotional rollercoasters that transition you from moments of hope to bouts of despair. These ups and downs are a natural part of recovery, reflecting the deep emotional scars left by manipulation, control, and dominance.

Periods of self-doubt may also emerge, where you question your worth or choices, feeling as though the ground beneath you is unstable. It's important to recognize that these feelings, while unsettling, are part of the healing process. They signal the mind's attempt to reconcile past experiences with present reality. Embracing these emotions with self-compassion can transform them from obstacles into stepping stones. Recovery is not about erasing the past, but integrating it into a healthier, more resilient self. Each emotion, whether painful or uplifting, is proof of your capacity to grow.

5.2 Stages of Healing

The stages of healing from narcissistic abuse unfold uniquely for everyone, often progressing in a non-linear fashion. As you embark on this journey, you may first encounter denial, a stage where you feel something is amiss but struggle to acknowledge its true nature. This phase can be a protective mechanism, shielding you from the immediate pain of recognition. As suspicions of abuse surface, they often lead to shock and confusion, where you grapple with the dissonance between perceived reality and the truth of your experiences. This cognitive dissonance can be disorienting, leaving you questioning your perceptions and memories.

As clarity begins to emerge, you enter the stage of identification, where you name and recognize the abuse for what it is. This stage is empowering, marking the beginning of reclaiming your narrative.

The separation stage often follows, involving a physical or emotional distancing from the abuser. This step can trigger a cycle of love bombing and rage from the narcissist, testing your resolve to maintain boundaries. Complicated grief often accompanies this separation, bringing with it emotions like anger, guilt, and sadness, all intertwined in a complex tapestry. This stage can be particularly challenging, as it involves mourning the relationship and the loss of what could have been.

Education becomes a powerful ally as you learn about narcissism and abuse, validating your experiences and finding support through self-help resources. The education stage fosters understanding, helping to dismantle the isolation that abuse often creates.

The recovery stage focuses on self-care, emphasizing the rebuilding of self-worth and independence. It's a time to nurture yourself and embrace activities that bring joy and fulfillment. Restoration involves reclaiming your independence and rebuilding your life based on personal values and goals. This stage is about constructing a future that reflects your true self, free from the constraints of past toxicity.

Next, the meaning-making stage emerges as you find personal growth from trauma, discovering resilience and healthier boundaries. This stage transforms pain into purpose, allowing you to redefine your narrative.

Paying it forward, the final stage, involves sharing your experiences to help others, providing a sense of closure and positive change. Giving back strengthens your own healing and contributes to the healing of others, creating a ripple effect of hope and empowerment.

Throughout this journey, remember that healing is possible. Each stage, while challenging, brings you closer to a life of authenticity and peace. There are many who have been on this journey who found strength in vulnerability and emerged more resilient than before. Their recovery testimonials serve as beacons of hope, illuminating the way forward. Let these words inspire you to embrace your journey, knowing that each step you take is a testament to your courage and determination.

Reflection Exercise: Mapping Your Healing Journey

Consider creating a visual map of your healing journey, marking significant events and emotional milestones. Use colors or symbols to represent different stages and emotions. Reflect on how far you've come and the progress you've made, acknowledging each step as a victory in itself.

5.3 Effective Communication Techniques

Navigating conversations with a narcissist often feels like walking a tightrope, where balance is key to avoiding a fall into conflict. Assertive communication stands as a vital tool in this delicate dance. It's about expressing your needs and feelings clearly, without aggression or submission. Using "I" statements can be transformative in these exchanges. Instead of saying, "You never listen to me," you might instead express, "I feel unheard when my words are interrupted." This subtle shift focuses on your experience rather than casting blame, reducing defensiveness and opening the door to more constructive dialogue. It's a way to assert your feelings while respecting the other person, fostering an environment where both parties feel acknowledged. By taking ownership of your emotions, you protect your self-esteem and invite the narcissist to engage in a more balanced interaction.

Conflict with a narcissist can escalate swiftly, often leaving you feeling overwhelmed and powerless. De-escalation techniques become essential in managing these situations. Keeping a neutral tone is one of the most effective strategies. When emotions run high, a calm and steady voice can defuse tension, signaling you're not engaging in a battle of wills. It helps maintain a level ground where discussions can happen without spiraling into arguments. Avoiding personal attacks is equally crucial. Instead of pointing fingers, focus on the issue at hand. Personal attacks only serve to entrench the narcissist in their position, making resolutions more elusive. By steering clear of accusations, you create space for dialogue rather than defensiveness, allowing for more productive conversations.

Active listening is another cornerstone of effective communication, often overlooked yet incredibly powerful. It involves listening to understand, not just to respond. Reflective listening techniques can aid in this process. By paraphrasing what the other person has said, you demonstrate that their words have been heard and understood. For instance, if someone says, "I feel like you're always busy," a reflective response might be, "It sounds like you're feeling neglected because I haven't been around much." This approach validates their emotions and clarifies misunderstandings. Active listening fosters a sense of being heard, which can alleviate some of the tension inherent in communicating with a narcissist.

Non-verbal communication can influence interactions in subtle yet profound ways. For example, your body language and facial expressions can impact how your message is received, reinforcing or undermining your verbal communication. Maintaining an open body posture is a simple yet effective way to convey receptiveness and willingness to engage. This includes facing the person directly, keeping your arms uncrossed, and maintaining an appropriate level of eye contact. These non-verbal cues signal that you are present and attentive, encouraging a more open exchange. Similarly, facial expressions can communicate empathy and understanding, softening the edges of difficult conversations. A nod or a gentle smile can show that you are engaged and empathetic, helping to build rapport even in tense situations.

Incorporating these communication techniques requires practice and patience. It might feel challenging initially, as old habits and patterns can be difficult to break. However, with time and persistence, these strategies can become second nature, equipping you with the tools to navigate difficult conversations gracefully and confidently. Remember, communication is not just about conveying your message; it's about creating an environment where understanding and respect can flourish. Effective communication transforms interactions, reducing conflict and fostering healthier, more balanced relationships. By embracing these techniques, you take a significant step toward reclaiming your voice and ensuring your needs are heard and respected.

5.4 Creating a Supportive Environment

Imagine your life as a garden, with each relationship being a different plant contributing to the ecosystem. Some plants nurture the soil, while others drain it. Building a strong support network means cultivating those connections that nurture you, allowing your garden to flourish. Being surrounded by people who understand and support you isn't just comforting; it's vital for your recovery.

Joining support groups can be an excellent way to connect with others who have had similar experiences. These groups provide a safe space to share your story without fear of judgment, where empathy and understanding are the norms rather than the exceptions. Reconnecting with positive influences in your life, those who knew you at your best, can also serve as a powerful reminder of your true self. These people can offer insights and encouragement, helping you rebuild the confidence and identity that may have been eroded over time.

Community engagement can further reinforce your support network. These platforms offer a sense of belonging, where you can exchange advice, share victories, and support others. The anonymity of online interactions can be liberating. In these communities, you'll find a wealth of shared wisdom and encouragement, reminding you that you are not alone in your journey. This collective strength can be a powerful motivator, inspiring you to continue moving forward, even when the road feels daunting.

Creating a positive home environment is equally important in fostering a sense of peace and healing. Your home should be a sanctuary where you can retreat from the outside world and recharge. Remove any items with negative associations or memories. A tidy, organized environment can improve your mental clarity and emotional well-being. Consider incorporating elements that promote relaxation and comfort, such as soft lighting, soothing colors, or calming scents. These small changes can transform your home into a haven of tranquility where you feel safe and supported.

In addition to physical changes, consider the emotional atmosphere of your home. Surround yourself with things that bring you joy and inspire positivity. This might include photographs of loved ones, artwork that speaks to your soul, or music that lifts your spirits. Creating a home that reflects your values and desires can reinforce your sense of identity, reminding you of the strength and resilience that reside within you. It's about creating a space that nourishes your spirit and supports your growth, providing a foundation for healing and renewal.

As you cultivate this supportive environment, remember it is an ongoing process. Relationships may evolve, and your needs may change over time. Be open to reassessing your support network and making adjustments as necessary. Prioritize connections that uplift and empower you, and don't be afraid to distance yourself from those that drain your energy. Your well-being is paramount, and creating a supportive environment is crucial in nurturing your emotional health and resilience.

5.5 Journaling for Personal Growth and Clarity

Imagine sitting quietly with a pen and notebook, your thoughts flowing onto the page. This simple act of journaling can become a powerful tool for self-reflection and emotional processing. It helps you to untangle complex feelings and gain clarity. It invites you to pause and reflect, understanding the swirling emotions that often feel overwhelming. As you write, you might uncover insights about yourself hidden in everyday life's chaos, providing you with a clearer understanding of your journey.

Even though I have mentioned journaling previously, this section will provide a more in-depth look at various methods that you can adopt that will suit you the best. You may want to use several of these methods. Experiment with each one to identify which one(s) are most helpful.

Reflective writing exercises can be particularly beneficial in this process. They encourage you to delve into specific emotions or experiences, prompting you to explore them in depth. These exercises might ask you to consider how a particular event made you feel or what lessons you can draw from a challenging situation. Prompt-based journaling offers structured guidance, helping you focus on specific areas of your life that may need attention. Prompts like, "What am I grateful for today?", or, "What challenges did I face, and how did I overcome them?", can guide your writing, providing a framework that encourages introspection and growth. Through these exercises, journaling becomes a record of your thoughts and a tool for transformation.

The benefits of journaling extend beyond the moment of writing. By regularly reviewing past entries, you can track your progress over time, observing how your thoughts and feelings evolve. This retrospective view can offer valuable insights into your emotional patterns and triggers, helping you identify areas where growth has occurred or where further work is needed. It allows you to see your journey in a new light, recognizing the resilience and strength that has carried you through difficult times. In moments of doubt, these reflections can remind you of your capacity for change and healing, reinforcing the belief that you are moving forward, even when the path feels uncertain.

Different journaling techniques cater to individual preferences and needs, ensuring the practice remains engaging and relevant. Stream-of-consciousness writing, for example, is a technique that encourages spontaneity and authenticity, capturing the raw essence of your emotions. It can be liberating to release your thoughts without the pressure of coherence or grammar, allowing your inner voice to speak freely. On the other hand, gratitude journaling focuses on acknowledging the positive aspects of your life. By listing things you are thankful for, you shift your focus from negativity to appreciation, fostering a more positive mindset. Both methods offer unique benefits, allowing you to explore different facets of your emotional landscape.

Incorporating journaling into your daily routine can be a powerful tool for ongoing personal growth. Setting aside dedicated time each day for writing creates a ritual reinforcing self-reflection's importance. Whether in the morning with a cup of coffee or in the evening as a way to unwind, finding a time that works for you ensures that journaling becomes a consistent part of your life. Consider creating a comfortable, distraction-free space for your writing, where you can focus on your thoughts and feelings. This dedicated time becomes a sanctuary—a safe space to explore your emotions and gain clarity.

As you embrace the practice of journaling, you may find that it becomes a trusted companion in your healing process. Putting pen to paper invites you to explore your inner world, uncovering insights and fostering self-awareness. It provides a record of your journey—a tangible representation of your growth and resilience. Through regular journaling, you cultivate a more profound understanding of yourself, building a foundation for continued personal development. This practice not only aids in processing past experiences, but also equips you with the tools to navigate future challenges with confidence and clarity.

In this chapter, we've explored practical strategies for coping and healing, from building emotional resilience to creating supportive environments. We've delved into the power of communication and the transformative potential of journaling. As we move forward, we'll uncover new ways to foster personal growth and resilience, drawing connections to our broader journey of healing and empowerment.

SUMMARY of CHAPTER 5

Stages of Healing

- Denial is a stage where you feel something is amiss but struggle to acknowledge its true nature.

- Name and recognize the abuse for what it is. This stage is empowering, marking the beginning of reclaiming your narrative.

- Self-help resources will help you learn about narcissism and abuse, validate your experiences, and find support.

- The meaning-making stage transforms pain into purpose. This stage emerges as you find personal growth from trauma, discovering resilience and healthier boundaries.

- Paying it forward involves sharing your experiences to help others, providing a sense of closure and positive change.

Strategies for Communicating Effectively

- Keeping a neutral tone is one of the most effective strategies. A calm and steady voice can defuse tension, signaling you're not engaging in a battle of wills.

- Active listening is incredibly powerful, as it involves listening to understand.

- Fully engage with the speaker by being attentive.

- Non-verbal communication includes facing the person directly, keeping your arms uncrossed, and maintaining an appropriate level of eye contact. Similarly, facial expressions can communicate empathy and understanding.

    - These non-verbal cues signal that you are present and attentive, encouraging a more open exchange.

Recommendations for Supporting Your Journey

- Community engagement can further reinforce your support network. Online forums and discussions provide a safe space to share similar experiences with others.

- Create a positive home environment to foster a sense of peace and healing:

    - Make physical changes by decluttering and organizing your space, removing items with negative associations or memories.

    - Change the emotional atmosphere of your home. Surround yourself with things that bring you joy and inspire positivity.

- Reassess your support network. Associate with individuals who uplift and empower you, and don't be afraid to distance yourself from those who drain your energy.

- Use journaling techniques:

    - Reflective writing exercises delve into specific emotions or experiences, prompting you to explore them in depth.

    - Prompt-based journaling offers structured guidance, helping you focus on areas of your life that may need attention.

- Stream-of-consciousness writing involves letting your thoughts flow freely onto the page without censorship or structure.

- Gratitude journaling focuses on acknowledging the positive aspects of your life.

Title: Your Voice Can Help Set Someone Free

Subtitle: A Simple Act of Kindness Can Light the Way

"You are no longer going to survive; you are going to thrive." — Joan Hannon

You've read the pages, taken in the lessons, and begun to break free from the chains of narcissistic abuse, emotional abuse, and toxic relationships. Now, imagine helping someone else take that first brave step toward freedom.

Many people struggling with mental and even physical abuse feel trapped, confused, and alone. They don't know where to turn or how to start their journey. That's where your voice can make a difference.

Why Your Review Matters
Books like *Escaping the Narcissistic Abuse Prison* don't just tell stories—they save lives. But most people decide which book to pick up based on what others say.

By leaving a review, you could:

- Help someone discover they're not alone.

- Offer hope to a person searching for answers.

- Guide a survivor toward healing and empowerment.

- Show someone that freedom from abuse is possible.

It's Quick, Free, and Powerful
Leaving a review takes just a minute, but the impact could last a lifetime for someone in need.

To share your thoughts and help another person find hope, simply scan the QR code below or visit the book's review page online:

https://www.amazon.com/dp/B0D92NFP1Y

Thank You for Being a Beacon of Hope
Every kind word you share sends ripples of encouragement into the world. Together, we can help more survivors escape the invisible prison of narcissistic abuse and reclaim their lives.

From the bottom of my heart, thank you for being part of this mission.

Warmly,
Joan Hannon

Chapter 6:

A Holistic Approach to Recovery

Imagine looking over a vast landscape, the horizon stretching endlessly before you. The view is both daunting and exhilarating, much like embarking on this journey to recovery from narcissistic abuse. This journey is not just about moving away from pain, but also about discovering new ways to heal and grow.

Therapy and professional help are critical in this process, offering structured support and guidance. Seeking treatment is a courageous step towards understanding and reclaiming your life. Professional support can provide the tools to process your experiences, change negative thought patterns, and build healthier coping strategies. This chapter explores the various therapeutic approaches that can aid your recovery, highlighting their benefits and how they can be integrated into your healing journey.

6.2 Exploring Various Therapeutic Approaches

Individual Therapy

Individual therapy sessions can serve as a sanctuary and provide guidance from a trained professional. Finding a therapist who specializes in narcissistic abuse recovery can make all the difference. They understand the nuances of such relationships and can help you navigate the emotions that arise. Therapy provides tools for coping and healing, assisting you in unpacking the layers of trauma and rebuilding your sense of self. It's a collaborative process where you and your therapist work together to address the challenges and celebrate the triumphs of your recovery. This professional support can serve as a stabilizing force, offering clarity and perspective when the path ahead feels uncertain.

Some techniques that a therapist might use include:

- Cognitive-behavioral therapy (CBT) treats the trauma associated with narcissistic abuse. CBT focuses on identifying and reframing negative thought patterns and can be transformative, shifting your perspective and empowering you to take control of your emotional responses.

- Eye movement desensitization and reprocessing (EMDR) involves guided eye movements to help you process and integrate traumatic memories, reducing their emotional impact. This technique can provide relief from anxiety and PTSD symptoms, offering a path to peace and clarity.

- Psychodynamic therapy offers a deep dive into understanding how past experiences shape present behavior. This approach focuses on the unconscious mind, exploring how unresolved conflicts and emotions influence your life. Each session unravels another layer of your psyche, revealing insights into patterns that may have formed long ago. This therapy is about making the unconscious conscious, helping you gain insight into your emotional world. It can be a profound experience, allowing you to connect the dots between your past and the challenges you face today

- Dialectical behavior therapy (DBT) is another approach worth considering, especially for those dealing with intense emotions. Developed to treat borderline personality disorder, it has also proven effective for a range of emotional issues, including the aftermath of narcissistic relationships. It combines cognitive-behavioral techniques with mindfulness practices, teaching you how to manage emotions and navigate relationships with greater ease. DBT focuses on building four key skills: mindfulness, distress tolerance, emotion regulation, and interpersonal effectiveness.

    o Mindfulness helps you stay grounded in the present moment, reducing anxiety about the past or future.

- Distress tolerance equips you with strategies for processing painful emotions without resorting to self-destructive behaviors.

- Emotion regulation teaches you how to change emotional responses that disrupt your life.

- Interpersonal effectiveness improves your ability to communicate and assert your needs clearly, fostering healthier connections.

By working through your experiences in therapy, you begin to understand the dynamics that have shaped your life and, more importantly, how to break free from them. I would highly recommend therapy once you free yourself from a narcissistic relationship. It can help you to navigate through the tangle of emotions that you are feeling and identify areas that may be more problematic than you realize.

There is so much confusion when you break free from the narcissistic prison and attempt to reclaim your life. Therapy can bring so much clarity and map out a path for you that may be harder to achieve when you are attempting to find your way alone through the maze of emotions. A good therapist will be able to assist you in taking the jumbled thoughts and confusion, helping you identify and address those emotions in a fashion that will allow you to heal much quicker. Having that one-on-one personalization provides comfort and security that you might not have otherwise.

Group Therapy

Group therapy offers a different but equally valuable form of support. In a group setting, you share understanding, empathy, and encouragement.

Sharing your story in a group can be empowering, serving as a reminder that you are not alone in your struggles. The communal aspect of group therapy fosters empathy and connection, allowing you to build relationships based on mutual support and respect. It's a space where you can practice new coping strategies and receive feedback in a safe, nonjudgmental environment. This shared journey can be incredibly healing as you witness the progress of others while celebrating your own milestones.

6.3 Finding the Right Therapist or Counselor

Finding the right therapist can feel like choosing the perfect pair of shoes—you need the proper fit. With so many therapeutic modalities available, it's important to consider what aligns best with your needs and personality.

When choosing a therapist, consider what resonates with you. Are you drawn to exploring the depths of your psyche, or do you prefer practical tools to manage day-to-day challenges? The therapeutic relationship is a partnership, and it is critical to find someone who you are comfortable with and trust. Don't hesitate to ask potential therapists about their approaches, and how they might tailor them to your specific situation. Remember, this is about your healing and growth; you have the right to seek what feels right for you.

Reflecting on what you hope to achieve in therapy can guide your decision. If you're unsure of where to start, consider what you want to change in your life and what support you need to get there. Sometimes, the process of finding the right therapist is about trial and error, and that's okay. Each step you take towards understanding and healing is a step in the right direction. Trust your instincts, and know that the appropriate support is out there.

Reflective Exercise: Exploring Therapy Options

Consider your personal needs and preferences when exploring therapy options. In your journal, reflect on the following questions to gain clarity on what might be the best fit for you:

- What are your primary goals for therapy? Are you looking to explore deeper emotional issues, or seeking relief from specific symptoms?

- Do you prefer one-on-one interactions, or feel more comfortable sharing experiences with a group?

- What are your feelings towards different therapeutic approaches like CBT or EMDR? Are you open to trying new techniques, or do you have previous experiences that guide your choice?

By reflecting on these questions, you can identify the type of therapy that aligns with your needs, setting the stage for a more tailored and effective healing process.

6.4 Building a New, Empowered Identity

Imagine standing in front of a blank canvas, ready to paint your life anew. This is the moment to explore new interests and redefine who you are, free from the shadows of past abuse.

Reclaiming your identity is not only possible, but is also necessary for moving forward.

Trying new hobbies or classes can be like adding vibrant colors to your world; each brushstroke is a step toward discovering passions that once brought joy and fulfillment. Whether it's learning to play a musical instrument, taking up pottery, joining a local book club, painting, writing, or any other activity that used to light up your life, these activities offer fresh perspectives and a chance to meet new people. They help you reconnect with your senses of joy and curiosity, reminding you that life is a rich tapestry waiting to be explored. By stepping into these new experiences, you begin to carve out a space where your identity can flourish. These interests can help rekindle a sense of purpose.

Personal values are the compass that guides this exploration. Aligning your actions with core values ensures that the path you choose is fulfilling and authentic to who you are. Identifying your values might involve reflecting on what truly matters to you, what principles you hold dear, and what you cannot compromise on. This clarity allows you to set value-driven goals, creating a roadmap that aligns with your deepest beliefs. Perhaps you value honesty, creativity, or community. Whatever your values, let them inform your decisions, shaping a life that feels right at its core. When your actions reflect your values, you build a life that resonates with your true self, fostering a sense of empowerment and purpose.

As you redefine your identity, consider strategies for self-empowerment that cultivate confidence and independence. Taking on leadership roles, whether in your community, at work, or through volunteering, can be transformative. These roles challenge you to step outside your comfort zone, and to lead with integrity and vision. They help build self-assurance, showing that you can make a difference and inspire others. Leadership is not about the title, but about action and influence. By taking initiative, you affirm your capability and reinforce your self-worth. Each experience strengthens your independence, allowing you to stand tall, knowing you have the skills and resilience to face whatever comes your way.

Celebrating individuality and uniqueness is key to embracing an empowered identity. Your unique traits and characteristics are not just aspects of who you are; they are your strengths. Personal style expression, whether through fashion, art, or lifestyle choices, is a powerful way to honor your individuality. It's about letting your true self shine, unafraid of judgment or conformity. This celebration of self allows you to embrace your quirks and talents, seeing them as assets rather than flaws. By valuing what makes you different, you cultivate a sense of pride and confidence in your identity. You realize your uniqueness is your superpower, offering perspectives and ideas that no one else can.

The journey to self-discovery is profoundly personal and uniquely yours. Though the path may be fraught with challenges, it is also one of empowerment and growth. Through self-reflection, reconnecting with your passions, and embracing your true self, you can emerge from the shadows of narcissistic abuse stronger and more resilient than before.

6.5 Embracing Change and Growth

Change is a constant, much like the seasons inevitably transition from one into the next. While it can be unsettling, embracing change opens the door to personal growth and transformation. Viewing change not as a disruption, but instead as an opportunity, can shift your perspective, allowing you to see new possibilities and potentials. Think of it as a chance to rewrite your story, to discard what no longer serves you, and to make room for something new and enriching. This mindset turns change into a powerful ally, guiding you toward a future that feels more aligned with your true self. Embracing change means welcoming the unknown with open arms, trusting that each shift brings lessons and opportunities for growth.

- Developing a flexible mindset is vital, allowing you to adjust your sails rather than resist the winds of change. Flexibility means being open to new ideas and ways of doing things, even if they initially seem challenging. It's about seeing setbacks not as failures but as stepping stones to learning and improvement.

- Continuous personal development lies at the heart of embracing change. Enrolling in educational courses can reignite your passion for learning, introducing new skills and knowledge that enrich your life. Whether it's a creative writing class, a digital marketing workshop, or a mindfulness course, education broadens your horizons and expands your potential.

- Setting personal growth milestones can also provide direction and motivation. These milestones are markers on your path, guiding you toward your goals and celebrating each achievement. They remind you of your progress, reinforcing your commitment to growth and transformation.

Reading stories of others' transformation can also offer inspiration and insight into powerful examples of how embracing change can lead to profound personal growth. For instance, consider the tale of a woman who decided to pursue her passion for art after years in a stagnant career. She enrolled in evening classes, dedicating herself to honing her craft. Over time, her work gained recognition, leading to exhibitions and a new career as a full-time artist. Her willingness to embrace change and step into the unknown transformed her life in ways she had never imagined.

Such narratives illustrate the growth potential within each of us, waiting to be unlocked by our openness to change. They remind us that transformation is possible and within our reach if only we dare to embrace the opportunities that change presents.

6.6 Mind-body Connection: Healing Through Movement

Imagine moving your body, the rhythmic flow of muscles and breath working in harmony. In its many forms, movement becomes a powerful ally in healing, offering benefits beyond the physical. Moving your body can improve your overall mood and release tension. Exercise also provides a sense of accomplishment, boosting your confidence and resilience.

Beyond the immediate emotional benefits, maintaining physical health contributes to overall stability, providing a strong foundation to tackle life's challenges. As you engage in physical activities, you may find that your energy levels increase and your outlook on life becomes more positive, empowering you to face obstacles with confidence.

Physical Activity

Exercise and physical activity are vital in reducing stress and enhancing mood, mainly due to the release of endorphins—as mentioned previously, those natural mood lifters flood your system during and after exercise. These endorphins act like a gentle balm, soothing stress and bringing a sense of happiness and well-being that permeates your day. You may find that regular exercise leads to improved sleep quality, helping your body recover and rejuvenate, and allowing you to wake up refreshed and ready to face the day.

Movement is more than physical; it becomes a pathway to deeper self-awareness. As you engage in physical activities, you connect with your body in ways that foster understanding and appreciation. Incorporating various forms of movement into your routine can enhance this mind-body connection, each offering its unique benefits:

- Yoga, with its calming effects, provides a sanctuary to find balance and serenity. The gentle flow of postures and the focus on breathwork create a meditative state, allowing you to release stress and cultivate inner peace. It encourages you to focus on each sensation, each stretch, and each breath. This heightened awareness cultivates a deep connection with your body, helping you recognize and release tension with intention. It's a practice of listening to your body's whispers, acknowledging its messages, and responding with care and compassion.

- Dance, on the other hand, becomes an expressive outlet, a way to communicate emotions and release pent-up energy. Whether it's a structured class or simply moving to music in your living room, dance invites joy and spontaneity, reconnecting you with the playful, creative aspects of yourself.

- Walking in nature, with its natural beauty and tranquility, becomes an exercise in mindfulness. As you walk, take in the sights, hear the sounds, and feel the sensations around you, grounding yourself in the present moment and finding solace in the simplicity of each step.

Walking in nature is my favorite method of physical exercise. I find that no matter how big a problem may seem before I take a walk, it is reduced to a much more manageable size by the time I return home. It is an exercise that most people can participate in. Even if you are unable to walk, getting outside on a warm sunny day will benefit you greatly.

Whether it's a morning yoga session, an evening dance class, or an afternoon walk, these activities become sacred time set aside for you.

Establishing a regular movement practice involves creating a weekly exercise schedule that aligns with your lifestyle and interests. This schedule becomes your commitment to self-care—a promise to prioritize your well-being. Over time, consistency leads to sustainable benefits, enhancing your physical health, boosting your emotional resilience, and deepening your connection with yourself. In this regular rhythm, you find the space to heal, grow, and embrace each day with renewed vitality.

Through mindful movement, you learn to honor your body's capabilities and limitations, embracing its unique rhythm as a source of strength and resilience.

6.7 Nutrition and Self-care as Healing Tools

Nutrition

Our body requires the right fuel to function at its best. Nutrition is pivotal in maintaining mental health, acting as a foundation for emotional and psychological well-being.

Tips for Eating:

- Listening to hunger cues is essential; it helps distinguish between physical hunger and emotional eating. This awareness can prevent the cycle of eating to cope with emotions, which often leads to guilt and further emotional distress.

- Mindful eating offers a pathway to healthier relationships with food, encouraging you to savor each bite and truly listen to your body's cues. The concept is simple yet transformative. It involves eating slowly, allowing you to appreciate the flavors and textures of your meals. By doing so, you enjoy your food more and give your body time to signal when it's full, preventing overeating.

Foods that assist in mood regulation and reduce symptoms of anxiety and depression:

Mindful eating fosters gratitude for the nourishment food provides, transforming mealtime into a nurturing ritual rather than a rushed necessity:

- Boost serotonin levels by eating foods such as bananas, oats, and turkey. These foods can elevate your mood and stabilize emotions. Serotonin, a neurotransmitter, is often referred to as the "feel-good" hormone. Its production is influenced by the intake of tryptophan-rich foods, which aid in mood regulation.

- Omega-3 fatty acids support brain health, and are found in walnuts and salmon. Omega-3 fatty acids are crucial for maintaining cognitive functions and reducing inflammation, which can affect mood and mental clarity. By including fatty acids in your diet, you give your brain the tools it needs to function optimally, reducing symptoms of anxiety and depression.

Staying Hydrated

Hydration is vital for maintaining overall well-being. Adequate water intake supports every cell in your body, from aiding digestion to regulating temperature. Staying hydrated can enhance concentration, improve mood, and prevent fatigue.

Dehydration can cause headaches and impair cognitive functions. Therefore, integrating enough water into your daily routine is crucial. As a reminder, drink regularly throughout the day. Hydration isn't just about quenching thirst; it's about sustaining the body's complex processes that keep you energized and focused.

Self-care

Self-care routines complement nutritional well-being by nurturing your mind and body. Self-care is not a luxury; it's a necessity for emotional nourishment. Incorporating self-care practices into your daily routine can aid in emotional recovery and resilience-building.

Some examples of self-care include:

- Skincare routines provide moments of relaxation and care, allowing you to connect with yourself in a tangible way. Taking time to cleanse, moisturize, and nurture your skin is not vanity; it's an act of self-love, reinforcing that you deserve care and attention.

- Relaxation activities are a vital aspect of self-care. Whether it's reading a book, soaking in a warm bath or hot tub, or taking a stroll in nature, these activities replenish your energy and restore your spirit.

- Relaxation techniques, such as aromatherapy, can enhance these routines. Aromatherapy uses essential oils to promote relaxation and emotional balance.
    - One of the ways I use aromatherapy is by immersing myself in a tub of hot water in which I have added scented Epsom salt, such as lavender or chamomile. I light a white candle, have soft spa music playing in the background, and burn an incense stick of lavender,

sandalwood, or frankincense. This is extremely relaxing and will detoxify your system. This is something you can do for yourself before going to bed as it will help you sleep soundly.

- Creating a calming evening routine can further enhance your well-being, preparing you for restful sleep and a fresh start each day. Consider incorporating soothing rituals, such as lighting a candle or playing soft music, to signal to your body and mind that it's time to unwind.

- Creative outlets for expression, such as painting, writing, or playing music, offer an additional avenue for self-care. These activities tap into your creative spirit, providing a sense of fulfillment and joy. As you engage in creative pursuits, you may discover new facets of yourself, building confidence and resilience along the way.

Self-care will impact emotional resilience, allowing you to recharge and face each day with renewed strength.

These practices create a sanctuary of peace and tranquility—a respite from the chaos of daily stressors. These routines serve as reminders that taking care of yourself is an ongoing practice that supports your journey toward healing and resilience.

6.8 Daily Practices for Emotional Resilience

Imagine waking up each morning with a sense of calm and clarity, ready to face the day with resilience and strength. Incorporate these daily practices for building emotional resilience and mental toughness.

Journaling

Even though I continue to mention journaling, I can't overstate the benefits of this activity. Disorganized, jumbled thoughts in our heads will keep us on a merry-go-round of confusion and helplessness. When you are writing your thoughts down, you will be amazed at how much clarity it can bring to why you feel the way you do. It will compartmentalize your thoughts in a way that will make sense, enabling you to act on those things that require action or leave those things alone that you can't control. I am always amazed at how many emotions will start pouring out as I start to journal. It's like talking to someone when you are attempting to solve a problem, and you will realize during the conversation that you have provided yourself with an answer to your own problem. This has happened to me innumerable times.

Keeping a daily gratitude journal can significantly enhance your emotional resilience. Each day, take a few minutes to jot down things you are grateful for. These entries don't have to be grand; they can be as simple as appreciating a cup of warm coffee or a friendly smile from a stranger. Over time, gratitude journaling can rewire your brain to seek out positivity, helping you build a solid foundation of emotional strength. As you cultivate gratitude, you may find that your challenges become more manageable as your perspective shifts toward one of abundance and possibility.

Writing down your thoughts and feelings allows you to explore who you are beyond the influence of the narcissist. It's a way to slowly piece together the fragments of your identity, acknowledging the pain but also celebrating the resilience that has brought you this far.

Take a moment to reflect on the activities and interests that once excited you. In your journal, create a list of hobbies or passions that were important to you before the relationship. Write about why you enjoyed these activities and how they made you feel. Consider how you might reintroduce them into your life, even if it's just a small step at first. Remember, this is about reclaiming joy and embracing who you are, free from external expectations.

Journaling and reflection provide a safe space to process emotions and gain clarity, helping you navigate complex feelings with understanding and compassion. Use your journal to explore your thoughts, fears, and aspirations, allowing your inner voice to express itself freely.

Managing Stress

Managing stress effectively is crucial for maintaining emotional resilience. Stress can creep in, often uninvited, disrupting your peace and clouding your judgment. Try the following techniques:

- Short breathing exercises can be incorporated into your daily routine. These exercises can be as brief as five minutes, where you sit quietly, bringing your attention to your breath. Notice each inhale and exhale, letting thoughts come and go without judgment. This practice anchors you in the present moment, creating a pause in the stream of constant thinking. You might notice that when you are stressed, you will breathe shallowly—almost holding your breath. This will hold tension in your body, whereas taking the time to become aware of your breathing will relax you almost immediately.

- Deep breathing exercises are a method used for stress management. When you find yourself overwhelmed, pause and take a few slow, deep breaths. Focus on the rhythm of your breath, allowing each exhale to release tension and each inhale to bring calm. This practice can help lower your heart rate and reduce anxiety, creating a sense of stability amidst chaos.

    - I start my day with Tai Chi Gung daily. It incorporates deep breathing throughout the routine. This is a gentle but effective practice that moves your body, but brings constant focus to your breath. This practice relaxes me greatly before I start my day. There are other breathwork techniques that you can use as well. Try different methods before settling on the breathwork practice that fits you best.

- Progressive muscle relaxation is another technique to consider, which involves tensing and then relaxing different muscle groups in your body. This exercise not only alleviates physical tension, but also fosters a sense of relaxation and tranquility, making it easier to cope with stressors.

6.9 Meditation and Mindfulness Practices

Consider practicing meditation, which invites you to pause and reconnect with yourself amidst the chaos of daily life. It's a tool for healing, offering mental clarity and emotional balance. When you meditate, you create a space where stress dissolves, and your mind finds a rare sense of calm. This calmness isn't just a fleeting moment; it becomes a foundation for building resilience.

With regular practice, meditation helps improve your focus and concentration, allowing you to navigate life's challenges with a centered and grounded presence. This clarity sharpens your awareness, enabling you to respond to situations with thoughtful intention rather than reactive impulse.

Meditation will also create space to listen to your inner voice and help you tune out the noise of the world, allowing you to focus on your true personal desires and goals. As you sit in stillness, consider what you want to achieve, what fulfills you, and what steps you can take to get there. This practice of self-reflection fosters clarity and intention, helping you align your actions with your values. It's about understanding not just what you want, but why you want it and how it aligns with who you are.

Meditation isn't one-size-fits-all, and various techniques cater to different needs and preferences:

- Guided meditation sessions offer a structured approach, where you follow a narrator's voice to explore themes like relaxation, gratitude, or self-compassion. This guidance can be exceptionally comforting if you're new to meditation, providing a gentle framework to ease you into the practice.

- Loving-kindness meditation focuses on cultivating compassion for yourself and others. This technique involves silently offering phrases of goodwill, such as, "May I be happy, may I be healthy," slowly expanding this kindness to encompass people in your life. This practice enhances empathy and fosters a deep sense of connectedness, reminding you of the shared human experience.

- Morning mindfulness meditation is one of the most effective ways to start your day. This practice involves dedicating a few moments to focus on your breath and center your thoughts. By doing so, you create a mental space free from the noise and chaos of daily life, allowing you to approach challenges with a clear mind.

Mindfulness meditation helps you cultivate awareness and presence, enabling you to navigate emotional turbulence with grace and composure. This practice encourages you to focus on the present, anchoring your thoughts and quieting the noise of anxiety. Starting a mindfulness practice can feel overwhelming, but it begins with simple steps.

You can extend these sessions after you have become comfortable with them, allowing this practice to become a natural part of your day. By setting aside time each day, you create a habit that nurtures your well-being, offering a refuge from stress and anxiety.

As you integrate meditation into your life, you'll find its effects ripple outward, influencing how you engage with the world. It enhances your ability to listen deeply to yourself and others, cultivating compassion and understanding. This mindfulness infuses your interactions with presence, allowing you to be more attuned to the needs and emotions of those around you.

Through meditation, you develop a toolkit for navigating life's challenges, knowing that you can return to this quiet space whenever needed.

Consistency is key to unlocking the full benefits of meditation. Establishing a daily meditation routine, even if brief, reinforces the practice. Consider setting a specific time each day to meditate, perhaps in the morning to start the day calmly or in the evening to unwind before sleep. A dedicated meditation space—a quiet corner with a cushion or chair—can also enhance your commitment. Over time, this routine becomes a cherished ritual—a moment of peace you look forward to. Meditation is about showing up for yourself, no matter where you are. This regular practice deepens the connection to your inner self, fostering resilience and clarity that extends beyond the meditation cushion.

As a personal example, I use sound meditation after I go to bed. This is the quietest part of my day, and I know I won't be interrupted. Doing meditation at this time relaxes me so that I can fall asleep easier. Using sound for meditation rewires your brain, syncing the two hemispheres together, and will benefit your happiness and inner peace. Investigate sound meditation to see if it might work for you. It was easier for me to use this method than the traditional method of quieting my mind.

No matter which method of meditation you use, it is a skill that takes time to develop. However, with practice, meditation can offer profound inner peace, clarity, and resilience. By centering your thoughts and embracing the present moment, you can create a mental space that is free from past hurts and future worries.

Gratitude

Practicing gratitude during transitions can also be transformative. By focusing on the positives, even in difficult times, you cultivate a sense of contentment and appreciation for the journey. Gratitude shifts your attention from what is lacking to what is abundant, fostering resilience and a positive outlook.

6.10 The Benefits of Being Alone

Taking time to be alone is not a traditional method of healing, and is not normally addressed. Once you leave an abusive relationship, you need to spend time with only yourself. It is a way to get in touch with your true self, reflect on your goals, and consider those things that bring you the most satisfaction and joy. You need time to get your bearings before moving forward. It's nice to have input from others, but we know best as to what brings us the most satisfaction and happiness. Our society encourages us to be involved and to stay busy. Staying busy without leaving yourself time to reflect becomes a distraction from focusing on the things that really matter. If you don't take time for yourself now, you will become busy with other things that will fill that void.

When I was widowed, I felt completely lost at first. I had spent so many years focused on my husband and his needs, as well as taking care of him in the last year of his life, that I had neglected my own needs. I realized I didn't know myself anymore. Even though I experienced loneliness those first couple of years, the alone time allowed me plenty of time to think and determine what I wanted for myself and my future. I truly did not know who I was, as I had immersed myself so completely in my husband's life, likes, and dislikes.

That alone time was incredibly valuable and healing for me. It gave me clarity that I wouldn't have had if I had attempted to distract myself with temporary fixes and busywork to forget my loss.

Even though the end of my relationship was due to my husband's death, the end of your narcissistic, abusive relationship will bring up the emotion of grief and you will experience all the stages of grief. Expect this, honor the emotions that arise, and give yourself all the time you can to process these emotions. In time, you will find yourself valuing your alone time and becoming very protective of that time.

Staying out of a romantic relationship as long as possible will also be beneficial, as it can become another distraction. You are at a vulnerable stage that requires inner reflection, and getting immersed in a close relationship at this critical stage will detract from your healing. You will put yourself in a position of focusing on another person once again and not focusing on yourself.

I know it is tempting to seek romance to fill the void you find yourself in, but it will not serve you at this critical juncture. You are vulnerable and will find that you have many trigger points that could negatively affect a new relationship right now. It would not be fair to you, or to your new romantic interest.

Get to know yourself thoroughly and heal so that you can move on with your life and embrace a loving, healthy relationship when the time is right.

SUMMARY of CHAPTER 6

Steps Toward Healing

Therapy

- Individual therapy provides structured support and guidance.

    - Cognitive-behavioral therapy (CBT) is used to treat the trauma associated with narcissistic abuse. CBT focuses on identifying and reframing negative thought patterns.

    - Eye movement desensitization and reprocessing (EMDR) is a powerful tool in processing trauma. EMDR involves guided eye movements to help you process and integrate traumatic memories, reducing their emotional impact. This technique can provide relief from anxiety and PTSD symptoms, offering a path to peace and clarity.

    - Psychodynamic therapy offers a deep dive into understanding how past experiences shape present behavior.

    - Dialectical behavior therapy (DBT) focuses on building four key skills: mindfulness, distress tolerance, emotion regulation, and interpersonal effectiveness.

- Group therapy provides a safe and supportive environment for sharing your experiences with others that have experienced similar experiences.

Rebuild Your identity

- Try new hobbies or classes.

- Align your actions with core values to ensure that your path is fulfilling and authentic to who you are.

- Implement strategies for self-empowerment that cultivate confidence and independence.

- Celebrating individuality and uniqueness is key to embracing an empowered identity. Your unique traits and characteristics are not just aspects of who you are; they are your strengths.

- Embrace change by welcoming the unknown with open arms, trusting that each shift brings lessons and opportunities for growth.

- Develop a flexible mindset by being open to new ideas and ways of doing things, even if they initially seem challenging.

- Continuous personal development involves a commitment to lifelong learning and self-improvement.

- Set personal growth milestones that mark your path, guiding you toward your goals and celebrating each achievement.

Exercise and Physical Activity

Exercise and physical activity are vital in reducing stress and enhancing mood, mainly due to the release of endorphins—those natural mood lifters that flood your system during and after exercise. Beneficial exercises include:

- yoga
- dance
- walking in nature
- swimming
- going to a gym
- hiking

Nutrition

Nutrition is also pivotal in maintaining mental health, and is a foundation for emotional and psychological well-being.

- Mindful eating offers a pathway to develop a healthier relationship with food.
    - Listening to hunger cues helps distinguish between physical hunger and emotional eating.
    - Boost serotonin levels by eating foods such as bananas, oats, and turkey.

- Omega-3 fatty acids reduce symptoms of anxiety and depression for brain health. These nutrients can be found in salmon and walnuts.

- Staying hydrated can enhance concentration, improve mood, and prevent fatigue.

Self-care Routines

- Cleanse, moisturize, and nurture your skin, reinforcing that you deserve care and attention.

- Try relaxation techniques, such as:

    - Read a book.

    - Soak in a warm bath.

    - Enjoy a quiet moment in nature.

- Creating a calming evening routine will signal to your body that it's time to unwind.

    - Light a candle.

    - Play soft music.

- Creating outlets for expression, such as painting, writing, or playing music, can offer an additional avenue for self-care.

Managing Stress

Meditation, or quiet reflection, creates space to listen to your inner voice. Try the following techniques:

- Short breathing exercises bring your attention to the present moment, and can be as brief as five minutes.

- Deep breathing exercises help to release tension and stress by focusing on the rhythm and depth of your breath.

- Progressive muscle relaxation can help relieve tension and relax your muscle groups

- Guided meditation can be particularly comforting if you're new to meditation.

- Loving-kindness meditation focuses on cultivating compassion for yourself and others.

- Mindfulness meditation centers your thoughts and embraces the present moment. This practice creates a mental space free from past hurts and future worries.

In addition to meditation, gratitude shifts your attention from what is lacking to what is abundant. Alone time will also help you regain your sense of self and heal your wounds.

Chapter 7:

Personal Stories and Testimonials

Imagine a ship caught in a storm, with the waves crashing relentlessly against its hull; the captain struggles to maintain control, the crew clings to hope amidst the chaos. This imagery mirrors the experience of navigating life after narcissistic abuse, where emotional tempests challenge your resolve and test your strength.

Survivors often face a myriad of obstacles, each demanding resilience and creativity to overcome. Emotional setbacks, like the relentless waves, can feel overwhelming. You might find yourself revisiting painful memories or doubting your progress. These setbacks are normal and part of the healing process, but they can also be disheartening.

Legal and financial issues often accompany the journey to recovery, adding another layer of complexity. Whether it's untangling shared finances, dealing with custody battles, or simply finding stable ground in the aftermath of an abusive relationship, these challenges require clear-headed problem-solving. Creative approaches become essential.

Take, for instance, the story of Sarah—a single mother who faced a custody battle with her narcissistic ex. She found support through a community legal aid service, which provided guidance and representation when she couldn't afford private counsel. She navigated the legal system by reaching out for help and securing a stable environment for her children. Her story highlights the importance of seeking resources and building a support network that offers practical and emotional assistance.

As you work through your own challenges, remember that resilience is not just about bouncing back; it's about adapting and growing despite adversity. It involves acknowledging setbacks without letting them define you. Building resilience often starts with small steps. You might focus on setting achievable goals, celebrating minor victories, and cultivating a mindset that embraces flexibility and change. These strategies help you weather the emotional storms, providing a foundation of strength and confidence that grows over time.

As a survivor, the power of creative problem-solving cannot be overstated. Consider the story of Alex, who faced financial instability after leaving an abusive relationship. Instead of feeling trapped, he explored freelance opportunities in his field, allowing him to stabilize his income while maintaining flexibility. This approach not only improved his financial situation, but also boosted his self-esteem and independence. Creative problem-solving enables you to tackle obstacles with a fresh perspective, turning challenges into opportunities for growth.

Perhaps the most profound lesson is the ability to view obstacles as opportunities. Every challenge is a chance to learn and grow, reshaping your narrative from one of victimhood to empowerment. When faced with setbacks, ask yourself: *What can I learn from this? How can this experience make me stronger?* Adopting this mindset transforms hurdles into stepping stones. It shifts the focus from what you've lost to what you can gain, fostering a sense of hope and possibility.

7.2 Learning From Others: Case Studies in Resilience

In the tapestry of human experience, stories of resilience shine brightly, illuminating paths once thought impassable.

Consider the case of Linda, who endured a decade-long relationship with a narcissistic partner. Her life was a series of controlled interactions; her self-worth was chipped away by constant belittlement and manipulation. Linda's journey towards recovery began when she realized she was not alone. She reached out to a local support group, finding solace in shared experiences. This network became a lifeline, offering empathy and understanding that she hadn't known in years. Through these connections, Linda discovered the power of collective healing, where each person's strength bolstered the next.

Therapy played a pivotal role in Linda's recovery. With the guidance of a compassionate therapist, she began to unravel the threads of manipulation that had entangled her mind. Therapy offered a safe space to explore emotions long suppressed, helping her rebuild her identity. The counselor introduced techniques like cognitive-behavioral therapy, which challenged negative thought patterns and fostered a healthier self-image. This therapeutic relationship was more than just sessions; it was a partnership in healing, where Linda learned to trust her own perception of reality. The process was transformative, enabling her to set boundaries that honored her newfound self-respect.

From Linda's story, several key takeaways emerge. First, the importance of support networks cannot be overstated. Whether through friends, family, or support groups, these connections provide a foundation of strength. They remind you that you are not isolated in your struggle, offering a chorus of voices that validate your experiences. Next, setting personal boundaries becomes a powerful tool for reclaiming autonomy. Linda learned to articulate her needs and limits clearly—a skill that initially felt daunting, but grew more natural with practice. Boundaries are not walls; they are guidelines that protect your well-being and foster healthier interactions.

The outcomes of Linda's resilience are evident in the life she has crafted post-recovery. Professionally, she pursued a career in social work, inspired by her own experiences to help others navigate similar paths. This new direction provided financial stability and a sense of purpose and fulfillment. Linda cultivated relationships built on mutual respect and understanding. She learned to trust again, albeit cautiously, and surrounded herself with people who valued her for who she truly was. Her journey is a testament to the human capacity for change, illustrating how resilience can lead to profound transformation.

Another case that highlights resilience is that of David, who spent years in a marriage marked by subtle undermining and emotional withdrawal. His partner's narcissistic tendencies left him questioning his worth, caught in a loop of self-doubt. The turning point came when David attended a workshop focused on emotional intelligence. There, he encountered concepts that resonated deeply, prompting self-reflection and growth. The workshop provided tools for recognizing and managing his emotions, empowering him to take control of his narrative.

The role of therapy further bolstered David's resilience. Engaging with a therapist helped him process the emotional scars from his marriage. They explored strategies for rebuilding confidence and self-esteem, gradually dismantling the belief that he was inadequate. Through therapy, David learned to forgive himself for past decisions, releasing the shame that had tethered him to his partner's criticisms. This process of self-acceptance was liberating, allowing him to embrace his own strengths and potential.

The lessons from David's journey emphasize the significance of self-awareness. By understanding his emotional triggers and responses, David regained control over his reactions, reducing the power his partner once held over him. This self-awareness extended to setting boundaries, a crucial step in his recovery. David's ability to establish firm yet compassionate limits prevented further emotional manipulation, creating a space where he could heal and grow.

The outcomes of David's resilience are seen in his renewed zest for life. He rediscovered hobbies that had been sidelined, finding joy in activities that nurtured his spirit. Professionally, David explored opportunities that aligned with his values, leading to a fulfilling career change. His personal life also flourished as he formed connections grounded in honesty and shared interests. David's story exemplifies how resilience can transform adversity into an opportunity for personal and professional growth, illustrating the profound impact of healing and self-discovery.

7.3 Shared Experiences: Community and Connection

In the wake of narcissistic abuse, finding a community that understands your experiences can feel like discovering an oasis in a desert. Shared experiences have a unique power to foster healing and support. When you connect with others who have walked a similar path, you realize you are not alone. This realization can be a lifeline, providing the validation and empathy that might have been missing in your life.

Participation in support groups offers a safe space to share your story and hear others' experiences, creating bonds that are both comforting and empowering. In these groups, whether online or in person, you will find people who speak your language, who nod in understanding as you recount the twists and turns of your journey.

Finding a supportive community provides both emotional and practical support, helping you navigate the complexities of healing. Online forums, for instance, offer a platform where you can share stories and seek advice from a diverse group of individuals. These forums create a sense of belonging as you engage with others who understand the nuances of narcissistic abuse. Local meetups for survivors offer another layer of connection, bringing together individuals in shared spaces to form real, tangible bonds. In these settings, you can look into someone's eyes and see a reflection of your own struggles and triumphs. The power of a community lies in its ability to transform isolation into solidarity, giving you the courage to voice your experiences and the strength to listen to others.

Through diverse community stories, you can witness the strength and solidarity that emerges from collective healing. Consider the story of a woman who, after years of silence, found her voice in a support group. Surrounded by others who had faced similar challenges, she was inspired to share her story for the first time. The group's response was overwhelming, offering validation and encouragement that fueled her healing process. Another individual, a man who had felt isolated in his experience, discovered an online community that provided support and became a source of lifelong friendships. These stories illustrate how community can be a powerful catalyst for healing, offering both a mirror and a window through which to view your own journey.

Building supportive networks is a crucial step in recovery. Many of these networks or organizations host events or workshops that provide opportunities to connect with others in similar situations. Online resources can also guide you to forums or virtual meetups tailored to your needs. When joining a new group, take the time to listen and observe, finding a space where you feel comfortable and safe. If you're inspired to start your own support network, begin by inviting a few trusted individuals to gather and share their experiences. Establish ground rules that prioritize respect and confidentiality, ensuring that all members feel secure and heard.

Through the power of shared experiences, you can find strength in connection. Being part of a community helps you realize that, while the path may be challenging, you don't have to walk it alone.

7.4 Triumph Over Trauma: Personal Narratives

Navigating through the aftermath of narcissistic abuse often feels like piecing together a puzzle with missing pieces. Yet, amidst the shards of past trauma, there are stories of individuals who have not only survived, but thrived.

Let me share the story of Emma, who once found herself shackled by the chains of emotional abuse. After escaping a narcissistic relationship, she felt like a shadow of her former self—her confidence and trust in tatters. However, the turning point came during a late-night conversation with a close friend. As Emma poured her heart out, she experienced an emotional breakthrough. This moment of vulnerability transformed into a catalyst for change, igniting a determination to reclaim her life. Emma embarked on a path of self-discovery, enrolling in therapy and slowly rebuilding her self-worth. Through this process, she learned to trust others again, forming relationships based on mutual respect and understanding.

Emma's journey from victimhood to empowerment is a testament to the resilience of the human spirit. By setting boundaries and embracing her newfound strength, she established healthy relationships that reflected her values. This transformation was not instantaneous; it required patience and self-compassion. Emma realized that her worth was not defined by the past, but by the choices she made in the present. Her story illustrates that empowerment is a deeply personal journey, marked by introspection and the courage to embrace change. As Emma found her voice, she also found a renewed sense of purpose. She began volunteering at a local women's shelter, sharing her experiences to inspire and support others. This newfound passion gave her life richness and fulfillment, proving that pain can be a powerful motivator for positive change.

Another inspiring narrative is that of Mark, who, after a decade of enduring subtle manipulation and control, decided to rewrite his story. For years, Mark felt trapped in a cycle of self-doubt—each decision overshadowed by the fear of disapproval. But one day, while attending a workshop on personal development, he experienced a shift in perspective. Surrounded by like-minded individuals, Mark realized that he was not alone in his struggles. This sense of community kindled a spark of hope, encouraging him to take control of his narrative. Mark's transformation began with small but significant steps. He started journaling his thoughts, a practice that helped him process emotions and track his progress. This self-reflection allowed him to identify patterns of behavior that no longer served him. Gradually, Mark built a new self-image, one rooted in authenticity and self-acceptance.

As Mark's confidence grew, so did his ability to form meaningful connections. He ventured into new social circles, seeking interactions that enriched his life. These relationships became a testament to his growth, each one reinforcing the belief that he was deserving of love and respect. Mark's journey emphasizes the power of self-awareness in overcoming trauma. By understanding his triggers and responses, he was able to navigate challenges with resilience and grace. His story is a beacon of hope, demonstrating that the path to healing is filled with opportunities for growth and transformation.

In these narratives, the steps and milestones of healing are vividly illustrated. Both Emma and Mark show that healing begins with acknowledging the pain and choosing to move forward. It involves embracing vulnerability and seeking support from trusted individuals. Through therapy, community, or personal reflection, each step forward is a testament to strength and a commitment to change. These stories remind you that, while the scars of trauma may never fully fade, they can become a testament to your resilience and capacity for growth.

The narratives of triumph over trauma serve as powerful reminders that healing is possible. They offer hope that your own story can be rewritten, filled with new chapters of courage, empowerment, and purpose. You are not defined by the experiences of the past, but by the choices you make today. As you read these stories, may you find inspiration to explore the possibilities that lie ahead and the strength to embrace the journey of healing.

7.5 Stories of Survival and Strength

Resilience is a thread woven through the fabric of survival, a testament to the human spirit's capacity to endure and thrive despite adversity. For many survivors, overcoming financial dependency is a significant milestone on their path to recovery.

Consider the story of Jane, who found herself financially tethered to a partner who used money as a means of control. After years of being told she couldn't manage on her own spending, Jane made the bold decision to take control of her finances. She enrolled in budgeting workshops, learned new skills, and found a job that provided financial independence and restored her confidence. Jane's resilience in overcoming financial dependency highlights the empowering effect of taking charge of one's life, proving that it's never too late to reclaim your power and autonomy.

The journey of a single parent like Lisa, who navigated the turbulent waters of independence after leaving an abusive relationship, serves as a beacon of hope for others. Lisa was initially overwhelmed, balancing work, childcare, and the emotional scars of her past. Yet, she tapped into an inner strength she didn't know she possessed. With the support of friends and community resources, Lisa managed to create a stable home environment for her children while pursuing further education. Her determination to build a new life from the ground up illustrates how resilience can transform daunting challenges into stepping stones for personal growth. Lisa's story is not just about survival; it's about redefining her life on her terms and providing a nurturing space for her family.

A survivor's journey post-divorce offers another powerful opportunity for rebuilding and renewal. Consider David, for example, who chose to start anew after leaving a manipulative marriage. The dissolution of his marriage was not just an end, but a beginning—a chance to rediscover his passions and redefine his identity. David found solace in creative pursuits, which became therapeutic outlets for processing his emotions. He also fostered new friendships that celebrated his authenticity. Through these connections, David realized that his worth was not determined by past relationships, but by his actions and choices moving forward. His story is a testament to the resilience of the human spirit, showcasing the ability to rise above past hardships and embrace a future filled with promise and potential.

Similar to David, another young professional named Alex embarked on his own path to self-discovery after leaving a toxic work environment. Alex faced a workplace marked by narcissistic leadership, where he constantly questioned his abilities. Leaving that environment was daunting, but opened doors to self-exploration and growth. Alex pursued interests that had long been dormant, taking courses that reignited his passion for learning. This journey of self-discovery enhanced his career prospects and enriched his personal life. Alex's narrative underscores the importance of listening to one's inner voice, and the courage it takes to pursue a path aligned with personal values and aspirations.

As each story demonstrates, inner strength is an essential element in navigating challenging situations—a quiet force that propels individuals forward, even when the path is unclear. This strength is often born out of necessity, emerging during moments of profound vulnerability. It's the determination to rise each day and face the world with resilience, despite the shadows of the past. For many survivors, tapping into this inner reservoir of strength is a gradual process. It involves acknowledging fears, embracing weaknesses, and recognizing their power within to overcome them. Whether it's through meditation, reflection, or the support of loved ones, accessing this inner strength allows survivors to navigate life's challenges with grace and fortitude. It's a reminder that, while the journey may be fraught with obstacles, the human spirit is capable of remarkable resilience and transformation.

7.6 Empowerment Through Others' Journeys

In the landscape of recovery, empowerment often emerges through the stories of those who have transformed adversity into triumph.

Consider the narrative of Maria, a once-unassuming individual who found her calling in the world of entrepreneurship. Her past was marked by the shadows of manipulation and control, yet she envisioned a future defined by independence and self-reliance. Maria's journey into business ownership was not a straightforward path; it was filled with moments of doubt and echoes of past criticism. However, she used these challenges as motivation to pursue her vision.

Maria began with a small idea—an online boutique that catered to unique, handcrafted goods. The initial steps felt daunting, but she leaned on her resourcefulness, drawing on her creativity and resilience to navigate the complexities of starting a business. Each sale, no matter how small, represented a victory over the voices that once told her she couldn't succeed. As her business grew, so did Maria's confidence. She found empowerment in the ability to make decisions and shape her destiny according to her own terms. Her success transcended financial gain; it was a testament to her ability to reclaim her narrative and build a life filled with purpose and autonomy.

Then, there's Rachel, a survivor who turned her experiences into a force for change. After enduring years of emotional abuse, she emerged with a profound understanding of the power of advocacy. Rachel discovered her voice while volunteering at a local shelter, where she offered support to others who walked similar paths. This work ignited a passion for activism, and she soon became a leading advocate for domestic abuse survivors in her community. Rachel's advocacy work expanded beyond the shelter. She began speaking at conferences, sharing her story to raise awareness and inspire others. Her words carried the weight of firsthand experience, resonating with audiences who saw in her a beacon of hope and resilience.

Rachel's journey is marked by a commitment to creating tangible change. She worked tirelessly to influence policy, collaborating with lawmakers to strengthen protections for survivors. Her efforts contributed to the implementation of new initiatives that provided resources and support for those in need. Through advocacy, Rachel found healing and empowerment, transforming her past pain into a powerful catalyst for social change. Her work uplifted others and reinforced her own sense of agency and purpose.

Both Maria and Rachel's stories highlight the transformative power of empowerment. They demonstrate how reclaiming control over one's life and using personal experiences as a platform for growth can lead to profound self-actualization. These narratives underscore the importance of pursuing passions that align with personal values, illustrating how empowerment can manifest in various forms. For Maria, it was entrepreneurship—a tangible representation of her independence. For Rachel, it was advocacy—a way to give voice to those who feel voiceless.

These stories serve as reminders that empowerment is not a destination, but a continuous process of self-discovery and growth. It's about finding the courage to step beyond the shadows of past experiences and into a future shaped by one's own hands. Whether through business, advocacy, or any other avenue, empowerment is about embracing the capacity to influence change, both within oneself and in the broader world.

As you reflect on these narratives, consider how the themes of empowerment and self-actualization might resonate with your own journey. You, too, have the power to transform past adversities into opportunities for growth and fulfillment. Empowerment comes from recognizing your strengths, pursuing your passions, and finding ways to contribute to your community and the world. The path may be challenging, but these stories show that it is possible to rise above and create a life that reflects your true self, free from the constraints of past abuse.

As you stay focused and committed to this path of healing and transformation, you will be able to add your success story to these and inspire others through your example!

Reflection Exercise: Turning Obstacles Into Opportunities

This exercise encourages you to see obstacles as opportunities for growth and self-discovery. Take a moment to reflect on a recent challenge you've faced. In your journal, write about the emotions it stirred and the steps you took to address it. Consider what you learned from the experience and how it influenced your perspective. Identify any positive changes that emerged as a result.

Personal transformation is a testament to the human spirit's capacity to adapt and thrive. Every roadblock provides an opportunity to rebuild, rediscover, and reclaim your life. You are capable of profound growth and change, and your story continues to unfold with resilience and hope.

Chapter 8:

Resources and Further Reading

Imagine finding yourself at the edge of a vast, uncharted ocean. You stand there, feet planted in the sand, and the horizon stretches endlessly before you. It's overwhelming, but there's also a sense of boundless potential; the possibility of connection and understanding. As you navigate your healing journey from narcissistic abuse, this ocean represents the vast resources and communities that await you. In this chapter, we will explore online support groups and communities which offer a lifeline of empathy, validation, and shared experience. These platforms are like islands in the ocean, with each offering a unique perspective and sanctuary where you can anchor your thoughts and emotions.

8.2 Online Support Groups and Communities

In this digital age, the opportunity to connect with others who understand your experiences is just a click away. Online support groups are an option for those recovering from narcissistic abuse. They provide a safe space to share your experiences, knowing you are not alone. One such platform is Reddit's "r/narcissisticabuse" community, a forum where individuals from around the globe gather to discuss their experiences, offer advice, and support one another. This community thrives on anonymity, allowing you to express yourself freely without judgment or repercussions. It's a place where your voice can be heard, and where you can listen to the voices of others who have walked a similar path.

Facebook also hosts numerous groups dedicated to narcissistic abuse recovery. These groups vary in size and focus, from broad communities that welcome anyone affected by narcissism to more specialized groups that cater to specific aspects of recovery. Joining a Facebook group can provide a sense of camaraderie and connection as you engage with other individuals who understand how complex narcissistic relationships can be. The discussions range from personal stories and coping strategies to questions about boundaries and self-care. Here, you can find both the comfort of shared experiences and the inspiration to move forward with your healing.

The benefits of these virtual communities extend beyond mere connection. They offer accessibility, allowing you to participate from the comfort of your home at any time that suits you. This flexibility means you can reach out when you need it most, whether it's the middle of the night or a quiet afternoon. Additionally, these forums provide diverse viewpoints, exposing you to a myriad of perspectives and insights that can enrich your understanding of your own situation. By interacting with a global community, you gain access to cultural and personal nuances that might otherwise remain hidden. This diversity can broaden your perspective, offering new ways to approach and process your experiences.

When choosing an online support group, it's important to evaluate its credibility and supportiveness. Start by checking the group's moderation policies. A well-moderated group ensures that discussions remain respectful and on-topic, fostering a safe environment for all members. Moderation can prevent harmful or triggering content from taking over, allowing you to focus on healing and growth. Reading existing members' feedback can also provide valuable insights into the group's atmosphere and effectiveness. Look for groups where members actively support one another, and where the focus remains on recovery and empowerment. This supportive foundation is critical in helping you feel safe and understood.

Active participation is key to getting the most out of these communities. Engaging in discussions, sharing your story, and offering support to others can be incredibly therapeutic. By participating in weekly discussion threads, you contribute to the group's vibrancy and vitality while providing encouragement to others who may be struggling with similar experiences. Also, it helps you to process your emotions. Your insights and reflections can offer hope and guidance, reminding fellow survivors that healing is possible. As you interact with others, you build a network of understanding and empathy, creating a community that nurtures resilience and growth.

Reflection Exercise: Finding Your Community

Take a moment to reflect on what you are seeking from an online support group. Consider the type of environment that would make you feel comfortable and supported. Write down your thoughts and criteria, such as anonymity, diversity, or specific topics of interest. Use this reflection to guide your search for a community that resonates with you. Remember, the right group can provide support, a sense of belonging, and validation on your path to healing.

These online communities serve as beacons of hope and connection in the vast digital landscape. They offer spaces where your experiences are acknowledged and your voice is valued. As you explore these groups, you embark on a journey of shared healing, where the collective wisdom and compassion of others become a part of your own recovery.

8.3 Workshops and Seminars for Continued Growth

Imagine stepping into a room filled with people who understand you, who have faced similar challenges, and who are now seeking the same healing and growth as you are. This is the magic of workshops and seminars: They offer a unique environment that fosters community and shared learning, where you can connect with like-minded individuals on a similar path to recovery. These gatherings provide knowledge and a network of support, offering opportunities to learn from others' experiences and share your own. The sense of camaraderie you'll find in these settings can be incredibly empowering, reinforcing the idea that you are not alone in your journey toward healing.

Educational seminars focusing on narcissistic personality disorder (NPD) provide understanding of the complexities of narcissism. Attending psychology conferences on personality disorders can offer a wealth of knowledge from experts in the field. These events often feature lectures and discussions led by psychologists and researchers who specialize in NPD, and can provide a comprehensive understanding of its dynamics and impact on relationships. By immersing yourself in these learning environments, you gain access to the latest research and strategies for dealing with narcissistic behaviors.

Personal development workshops are another avenue to explore. These workshops often focus on building self-esteem, improving communication skills, and fostering emotional resilience—key components in healing from narcissistic abuse. Assertiveness training workshops, for example, can teach you ways to express your boundaries and needs effectively, empowering you to stand firm during your interactions with others. These sessions are designed to build confidence, helping you recognize your worth and assert your rights in any relationship. Equipping yourself with these tools lays the groundwork for healthier, more fulfilling connections in the future.

When searching for workshops and seminars, selecting those that align with your recovery goals is crucial. Start by checking the credentials of the speakers or facilitators. A reputable event will feature experts with a proven track record in their field, ensuring that the information you receive is both reliable and insightful. Reading past attendee reviews can also provide valuable insights into the event's effectiveness and relevance. These reviews will help you become informed as to which events will best support your healing journey.

Visualizing yourself in these learning environments can be a powerful motivator. Picture the energy and enthusiasm of a room filled with individuals committed to growth and understanding. Consider the potential for new friendships and connections with people who share your experiences and aspirations. These relationships can become a vital part of your support network, providing encouragement and accountability as you continue to heal and grow. The collective wisdom and diverse perspectives you'll encounter in these settings can offer fresh insights and inspiration, guiding you toward new paths of personal development.

Attending workshops and seminars is about more than just acquiring knowledge. As you engage with these communities, you will open yourself to a world of possibilities and connections that can enrich your life in meaningful ways. You are not alone, and through these shared experiences, you can find the strength and resilience needed to reclaim your life and forge a brighter future.

8.4 Recommended Books and Articles

Diving into a good book can be like finding a trusted friend who understands your experiences and offers comfort and guidance. When it comes to understanding narcissistic personality disorder (NPD) and the path to recovery, the right book can illuminate the journey, providing both insight and hope. *The Narcissist You Know* by Joseph Burgo is one such book. It delves into the various faces of narcissism, offering a detailed look at how these behaviors manifest in everyday life. Burgo's work helps demystify the complex nature of narcissism, arming you with the knowledge to recognize these traits in those around you and, perhaps, within yourself. His compassionate and clear writing style will help you to understand the impact of narcissism on relationships (Burgo, 2015).

Another seminal work is *Will I Ever Be Good Enough?* by Karyl McBride. McBride, a therapist herself, provides a roadmap for recovering from a narcissistic mother's emotional abuse. Her insights are both professional and personal, offering a combination of therapeutic strategies and empathetic understanding. This book is particularly poignant for those who may have spent a lifetime seeking approval and validation, helping to break the cycle of self-doubt and foster a sense of self-worth independent of external validation (McBride, 2008).

In addition to these books, articles from reputable sources offer fresh perspectives and in-depth analysis of NPD. "Understanding Narcissistic Personality Disorder" from the Lindner Center of HOPE (2014) is an excellent starting point for those seeking a concise yet thorough overview of the disorder. This article explores the diagnostic criteria, potential causes, and treatment options for NPD, providing a solid foundation for further exploration. Reading articles like this can help clarify concepts and offer a more comprehensive understanding of how narcissistic behaviors impact mental health and relationships.

Memoirs and personal narratives provide a deeply personal glimpse into the realities of living with and overcoming narcissistic abuse. *Educated* by Tara Westover is a powerful memoir that, while not solely focused on narcissism, touches on themes of control, manipulation, and the struggle for autonomy. Westover's story of breaking free from an oppressive environment to pursue her education is both inspiring and relatable for anyone who has felt trapped by the influence of a controlling figure. Her narrative highlights the resilience of the human spirit and the transformative power of education and self-discovery (Westover, 2018).

To gain a richer understanding of the psychological and emotional landscape shaped by narcissism, it is important to consider diverse perspectives. *Healing the Shame that Binds You* by John Bradshaw addresses the pervasive impact of shame, a common byproduct of narcissistic abuse. Bradshaw's work offers insights into how shame can be internalized and manifest in various aspects of life, providing practical strategies for healing and reclaiming personal power. This book emphasizes the importance of self-compassion and forgiveness in healing, encouraging readers to release the burden of shame and embrace their inherent worth (Bradshaw, 1988).

These resources collectively offer a tapestry of insights and experiences that can aid in your understanding of narcissism and its effects. They serve as companions on your path toward healing, providing both knowledge and empathy. By engaging with these works, you open yourself to new ideas and perspectives—each contributing to a more in-depth understanding of yourself and the dynamics of the relationships that shape your life. The stories and insights found within these pages can offer solace and strength, reminding you that you are not alone, no matter how challenging the road may seem.

8.5 Tools for Ongoing Self-improvement

Digital apps and platforms offer a wealth of resources to support and enhance your self-improvement journey, providing structure and guidance at your fingertips. One popular app is Headspace, known for its mindfulness and meditation programs. Whether you're a beginner or a seasoned practitioner, Headspace offers guided sessions that help cultivate calmness and focus, essential for managing stress and improving mental clarity. It's like having a meditation coach in your pocket, ready to assist you whenever needed.

Similarly, Moodpath is an app designed to help you track your emotional health. By prompting you to reflect on your mood and thoughts, it assists in identifying patterns that might go unnoticed in the hustle of daily life. This insight can be invaluable in understanding triggers and responses, empowering you to make informed choices about your well-being. Over time, you'll notice trends and shifts, helping you address issues as they arise. These tools are more than just apps; they become companions on your path to self-discovery and emotional resilience, offering support and insight at every step.

Educational platforms like Coursera and Skillshare also provide opportunities to expand your knowledge and skills. Coursera offers classes on a wide range of topics, including psychology, which can deepen your understanding of human behavior and relationships. Engaging in these courses can enrich your perspective and provide new strategies for managing interactions and building healthier connections. Skillshare caters to those who wish to explore creative pursuits, offering lessons in everything from photography to graphic design. Engaging with these platforms fuels your intellectual curiosity and creativity, fostering a sense of accomplishment and personal growth. Whether you're learning a new language or exploring digital art, these courses offer a structured yet flexible way to enhance your skills and passions.

For those who prefer a more tactile approach, journals and planners serve as valuable tools for organizing thoughts and setting personal goals. Bullet journals combine creativity with functionality, allowing you to track habits, plan your day, and reflect on your experiences in a way that resonates with your personal style. These journals provide a blank canvas where you can document your journey, celebrate achievements, and explore your inner world. Writing can offer clarity and insight that digital tools sometimes lack. As you chart your progress, you will create a tangible record of your growth, reinforcing your commitment to self-improvement.

Integrating these tools into your daily life requires intention and consistency. Setting daily reminders for app usage can help establish a routine, ensuring that self-care remains a priority amidst your responsibilities. For instance, you might schedule a meditation session with Headspace each morning, or set aside a few minutes each evening to log your thoughts in Moodpath. These small, regular practices can have a profound impact over time, gradually shifting your mindset and enhancing your emotional resilience. Similarly, carving out time each week for online courses or creative pursuits allows you to delve deeper into topics that interest you, fostering a sense of fulfillment and knowledge.

When it comes to journals and planners, consider setting aside a specific time each day to jot down your thoughts or plan out your goals. Whether it's during your morning coffee or before bed, this practice can ground you, providing a moment of reflection and calm. As you engage with these tools, remember that the goal is not perfection, but progress. Embrace the process, celebrate small victories, and grow at a comfortable pace. These resources are here to support you, offering guidance, support, and encouragement as you navigate the complexities of personal development.

8.6 Crafting Your Personal Healing Plan

Creating a personal healing plan can be likened to charting your own course across an ocean, where the destination is your emotional well-being and fulfillment. The process begins with identifying key areas for growth, akin to marking the points of interest on your map. These areas might include building stronger boundaries, enhancing self-esteem, or learning to manage stress more effectively. It's about acknowledging where you stand and deciding where you want to be. Determine your challenges and aspirations. Doing so lets you pinpoint specific aspects of your life that require attention and nurturing. This clarity lays the foundation for setting achievable milestones, which serve as the stepping stones to guide you toward your goals. These milestones should be realistic and attainable, ensuring that each step forward boosts your confidence and reinforces your commitment to healing.

As you outline these milestones, remember the importance of flexibility. Life is unpredictable, and your circumstances may change unexpectedly. Your healing plan should be adaptable, allowing you to adjust your path as needed. Periodic reviews of your plan can help you assess your progress and make necessary adjustments. This flexibility ensures that your plan remains relevant and effective, supporting your growth even when faced with unforeseen challenges. It's about understanding that healing is not a linear process, and that being open to change can lead to unexpected opportunities for growth. This adaptability empowers you to remain resilient and focused, even when the seas become rough.

Another crucial element of a successful healing plan is accountability. Sharing your plan with a trusted friend or therapist can provide the support and encouragement needed to stay on track. Regular check-ins with this support person create a sense of responsibility, motivating you to follow through on your commitments. These check-ins offer an opportunity to celebrate successes, discuss setbacks, and refine your strategies. They serve as a reminder that you are not alone in this process, and that others are invested in your well-being. This shared purpose reinforces the notion that healing is a collective effort, not a solitary pursuit.

To help you get started, consider using templates and examples as inspiration for crafting your own healing plan. An example daily routine for emotional well-being might include mindfulness meditation in the morning, a gratitude journaling practice at midday, and a reflective evening walk. These activities provide structure and routine, supporting your emotional health while promoting mindfulness and self-awareness. As you build your plan, tailor these suggestions to fit your unique needs and preferences. This personalization ensures that your plan resonates with your goals and values, making it more likely that you'll stick with it over time.

Crafting a personal healing plan is empowering. It's a declaration of your intention to prioritize your well-being and take control of your recovery. As you work through this process, you will have a deeper understanding of yourself and needs, providing meaningful growth and transformation. Your healing plan becomes a living document, evolving with you as you progress. It offers a sense of direction and purpose, providing a roadmap that guides you toward the life you envision for yourself.

Engaging with these strategies and resources lays the groundwork for a more resilient and fulfilling future. Each step you take brings you closer to a place of healing and empowerment, where you can thrive beyond the shadows of past trauma. As you continue to explore these paths, remember that healing is a journey of self-discovery that allows you to embrace your strengths and celebrate your progress along the way. This chapter has provided a framework for crafting a personal healing plan, illuminating the path forward with hope and determination. Now, as you continue to explore the resources and strategies available to you, may you find strength in the knowledge that healing is within your reach and that you have the power to shape your own future.

SUMMARY of CHAPTER 8

Resources for Your Journey

Online Support Groups and Community

- Reddit's "r/narcissisticabuse" community
- Facebook

Workshops and Seminars

- educational seminars
- personal development workshops
- assertiveness training workshops

Books and Articles

- *The Narcissist You Know* by Joseph Burgo
- *Will I Ever Be Good Enough?* by Karyl McBride
- "Understanding Narcissistic Personality Disorder" from Lindner Center of HOPE
- *Educated* by Tara Westover
- *Healing the Shame that Binds You* by John Bradshaw

Apps

- Headspace offers guided sessions that help cultivate calmness and focus
- Moodpath is an app designed to help you track your emotional health

Educational Platforms

- Coursera offers classes on a wide range of topics
- Skillshare is for those who wish to explore creative pursuits

Journals and Planners

- Bullet journals combine creativity with functionality

- Writing can offer clarity and insight that digital tools sometimes lack.

Conclusion

You are no longer going to survive; you are going to thrive. —Joan Hannon

As you reach the final pages of this book, take a moment to reflect on the journey we've shared. Together, we've explored the complex world of narcissistic personality disorder and its profound impact on relationships. We've delved into the emotional aftermath of narcissistic abuse, acknowledging the pain and confusion it often leaves in its wake. This journey was not just about understanding, but also about empowering you to rebuild your self-worth and break free from toxic patterns. We've navigated practical strategies and embraced holistic healing approaches to guide you toward a more fulfilling life.

You have been handed all the tools you need to break free from this prison. I have absolute faith in you and your ability to live a life of freedom and purpose. Victory over your abuser will come as you take one step at a time toward freedom. Can you taste freedom as you formulate your escape plan? It should be so tangible that you can put yourself there just by thinking about it.

Knowledge is a powerful ally on this path. By recognizing the traits and behaviors associated with narcissism, you've taken the first step toward awareness and recovery. Understanding these red flags helps protect you from further harm. Setting boundaries is essential. It's about reclaiming your space and ensuring you have the freedom to heal and grow. The no-contact rule, though challenging, is a tool for liberation. It allows you to distance yourself from toxicity and focus on your own well-being.

Breaking free from these patterns is vital. Toxic relationships can become a cycle, but you have the power to stop it. The strategies outlined in this book encourage you to rebuild your self-esteem and confidence. Rediscovering your identity involves embracing vulnerability and celebrating even the smallest victories. These steps are crucial in redefining your self-worth and carving out a life that reflects your true self.

Healing from narcissistic abuse requires a comprehensive approach. Your healing journey involves not just the emotional and psychological aspects, but also the physical. Movement, nutrition, therapy, and mindfulness all play a role in fostering holistic recovery. Each of these elements contributes to your overall well-being, helping you build resilience and strength.

Now, as you stand on the brink of transformation, I urge you to apply these strategies in your own life. Take action! Seek out additional resources and connect with communities that offer understanding and support. You are not alone on this journey. Many have walked this path before you, and many will walk it alongside you. Remember the personal stories and testimonials shared in these pages. They are testaments to the resilience and empowerment that come from overcoming adversity.

Hope and resilience are central themes across every chapter. Recovery from narcissistic abuse is not just possible; it is within your grasp. Believe in your strength and capacity for growth. The road may be long, but with each step, you move closer to a life free from the narcissistic prison and the shadows of the past.

I want to express my deepest gratitude to you for embarking on this journey with me. Your courage and resilience are inspiring. Healing is not easy, but your determination to confront and overcome the effects of narcissistic abuse is a testament to your strength. Remember, you are not alone. You have the support of those who understand your journey and the resources to help you succeed.

As you move forward, carry with you the lessons learned, and the hope instilled. Embrace the new possibilities ahead. You are capable of profound transformation and growth. Let this be the beginning of a new chapter, one filled with empowerment, healing, and joy. Thank you for allowing me to be a part of your journey, and know that I am here, cheering you on every step of the way.

Sharing Your Journey to Freedom

Now that you've taken the first steps toward breaking free from the narcissistic abuse prison, you hold a powerful gift: the wisdom and strength gained along the way. Your story matters and sharing it could light the path for someone still searching for answers.

By leaving an honest review of *Escaping the Narcissistic Abuse Prison* on Amazon, you can help others who are trapped in confusion and pain discover the guidance they need. Your review could be the sign they've been waiting for—the moment they realize they're not alone and that healing is possible.

By leaving a review, you could:

- Help someone discover they're not alone.

- Offer hope to a person searching for answers.

- Guide a survivor toward healing and empowerment.

- Show someone that freedom from abuse is possible.

Every kind word you share sends ripples of encouragement into the world. Together, we can help more survivors escape the invisible prison of narcissistic abuse and reclaim their lives.

To share your thoughts and help another person find hope, simply scan the QR code below or visit the book's review page online:

https://www.amazon.com/dp/B0D92NFP1Y

From the bottom of my heart, thank you for being part of this mission. You are a gift and treasure for this world!

Warmly,

Joan Hannon

It's been a long journey of courage, stamina, and resilience, but you are now standing at the mountain's summit, celebrating your remarkable and life-changing achievements!

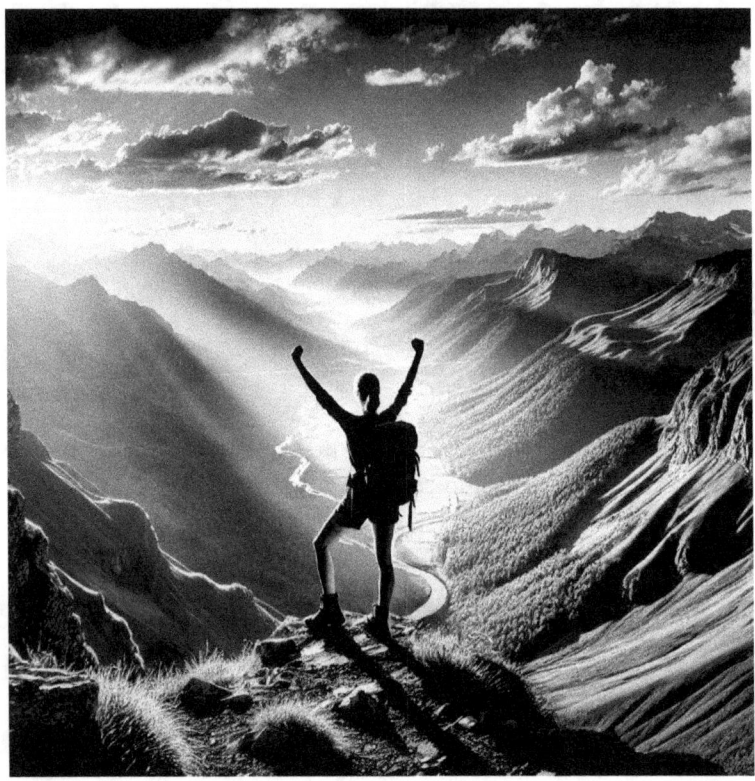

Glossary

Affirmations: Positive statements or phrases used to challenge and overcome negative thoughts and encourage self-empowerment.

Aromatherapy: The use of essential oils from plants to improve physical and emotional well-being.

Autonomy: The ability to make one's own decisions independently, maintaining a sense of self-governance.

Blame Shifting: A manipulation tactic where responsibility for a problem is transferred from one person to another.

Boundary Setting: Establishing clear limits to protect one's emotional and mental well-being.

Cognitive Restructuring: A therapeutic technique aimed at identifying and challenging distorted thought patterns.

Cognitive-Behavioral Therapy: A structured, goal-oriented type of psychotherapy that focuses on changing negative patterns of thought and behavior.

Covert Narcissism: A form of narcissism characterized by introversion, hypersensitivity, and a sense of victimization.

Codependency: A relational dynamic where one person prioritizes the needs of another over their own, often to an unhealthy degree.

De-escalation Techniques: Strategies used to reduce tension and prevent conflict from escalating.

Devaluation Phase: A stage in toxic relationships where one partner begins to belittle or demean the other after a period of idealization.

Deep Breathing Exercises: Techniques that involve slow, deliberate breathing to promote relaxation and reduce stress.

Discard Phase: The stage in a toxic relationship where one partner abruptly ends the relationship, often without explanation.

Dialectical Behavior Therapy: A form of therapy combining cognitive-behavioral techniques with mindfulness practices to address emotional regulation.

Emotional Abuse: A type of abuse that involves the use of words, behaviors, or actions to manipulate, control, or demean another person. This may include verbal insults, humiliation, threats, isolation, and other tactics intended to damage the victim's emotional well-being.

Emotional Manipulation: The use of deceit, guilt, or other tactics to control or influence another person's emotions.

Empathy: The ability to understand and share the feelings of others.

Emotional Abuse: A type of abuse that involves the use of words, behaviors, or actions to manipulate, control, or demean another person. This may include verbal insults, humiliation, threats, isolation, and other tactics intended to damage the victim's emotional well-being.

Empowerment: The process of gaining confidence and control over one's own life.

Eye Movement Desensitization and Reprocessing (EMDR): A therapeutic technique that helps individuals process traumatic memories using guided eye movements.

Gaslighting: A form of psychological manipulation aimed at making someone doubt their perceptions or sanity.

Genetic Predispositions: The inherited genetic traits that may influence an individual's likelihood of developing certain behaviors or conditions.

Grey Rock Method: A strategy to minimize interactions with manipulative individuals by becoming emotionally unresponsive.

Guided Meditation: A meditation practice led by an instructor or recording to assist with relaxation and focus.

Idealization Phase: The initial stage in a toxic relationship where one partner excessively admires and praises the other.

Insecurity: A feeling of uncertainty or lack of confidence in oneself.

Inner Child Healing: Therapeutic work aimed at addressing and resolving past childhood traumas or unmet needs.

Loving-kindness Meditation: A meditation practice focused on cultivating compassion and goodwill towards oneself and others.

Mean-making: The process of assigning personal significance to experiences, especially during difficult or transformative times.

Meditation: A practice of focusing the mind to achieve mental clarity and emotional calmness.

Mind-body Connection: The interrelationship between one's mental and physical health.

Mindful Eating: The practice of eating with full attention to the experience, focusing on the taste, texture, and sensations of food.

Mindfulness Practices: Techniques that promote present-moment awareness and reduce stress.

Morning Mindfulness: A daily practice of beginning the day with mindfulness exercises to set a positive tone.

Narcissistic Abuse: A form of emotional or psychological abuse inflicted by someone with narcissistic traits or Narcissistic Personality Disorder. This type of abuse may include manipulation, gaslighting, criticism, and control tactics designed to undermine the victim's confidence and sense of reality.

Narcissistic Personality Disorder (NPD): A mental health condition characterized by patterns of grandiosity, a need for admiration, and a lack of empathy. Individuals with NPD often have an inflated sense of self-importance and may exploit others to achieve their own goals.

Narcissistic Rage: Intense anger or aggression exhibited by a narcissist when their self-esteem is threatened.

No-contact Rule: A strategy to cut off all communication with a toxic individual to promote healing and recovery.

Omega-3 Fatty Acids: Essential fats found in foods like fish and nuts, beneficial for brain and heart health.

Overt Narcissism: A form of narcissism characterized by arrogance, attention-seeking, and entitlement.

Paying It Forward: The act of performing a kind deed for others in return for kindness received.

Physical Abuse: The use of physical force with the intent to harm, injure, or control another person. This includes hitting, slapping, pushing, choking, or other acts of violence that cause physical pain or injury.

Progressive Muscle Relaxation: A relaxation technique involving the tensing and relaxing of muscle groups to reduce stress.

Projection: A defense mechanism where one attributes their own thoughts, feelings, or traits to another person.

Prompt-based Journaling: Writing exercises guided by specific prompts to explore thoughts and emotions.

Psychodynamic Therapy: A therapeutic approach focusing on unconscious processes and unresolved past conflicts.

Reflective Writing Exercises: Writing practices used to examine and understand one's thoughts and experiences.

Repertoire: A range of skills, behaviors, or techniques available for use.

Resilience: The ability to recover quickly from adversity or difficulties.

Self-awareness: The conscious knowledge of one's own character, feelings, and behaviors.

Self-doubt: A lack of confidence in one's abilities or decisions.

Self-esteem: One's overall sense of self-worth or personal value.

Self-image: The mental picture or perception one has of themselves.

Self-worth: A sense of one's inherent value or worth as a person.

Serotonin: A neurotransmitter that contributes to feelings of well-being and happiness.

Shaming: The act of making someone feel humiliated or embarrassed, often used as a manipulative tactic.

Short Breathing Exercises: Quick and simple breathing techniques to calm the mind and body.

Smear Campaign: A deliberate effort to damage someone's reputation through lies or exaggeration.

Stream of Conscious Writing: A journaling technique where one writes continuously without concern for structure or grammar.

Visualization Techniques: The practice of imagining specific goals or scenarios to enhance motivation and focus.

References

American Psychological Association. (2019, October 30). *Mindfulness meditation: A research-proven way to reduce stress.* American Psychological Association. https://www.apa.org/topics/mindfulness/meditation

Bay Area CBT Center. (2024, July 8). *Distinguishing between overt vs covert narcissism.* Bay Area CBT Center. https://bayareacbtcenter.com/overt-vs-covert-narcissism/

Basyooni, A. (2024, July 4). *Overcoming isolation in a narcissistic relationship.* Circles. https://circlesup.com/blog/overcoming-isolation-in-a-narcissistic-relationship

Bradshaw, J. (1988, October 1). *Healing the shame that binds you.* Health Communications Inc.

Burgo, J. (2015, September 15). *The narcissist you know: Defending yourself against extreme narcissists in an all-about-me age.* Touchstone.

Caspari, J. (2023, May 7). *Embracing vulnerability.* Psychology Today. https://www.psychologytoday.com/us/blog/living-well-when-your-body-doesnt-cooperate/202305/embracing-vulnerability

Co-parenting with a narcissist: Tips and strategies. (n.d.). Custody X Change. https://www.custodyxchange.com/topics/custody/special-circumstances/co-parenting-with-narcissist.php

Cuncic, A. (2023, November 6). *Effects of narcissistic abuse*. Verywell Mind. https://www.verywellmind.com/effects-of-narcissistic-abuse-5208164

Dorwart, L. (2024, September 13). *The best mental health apps, tried and tested*. Verywell Mind. https://www.verywellmind.com/best-mental-health-apps-4692902

Exercise and mental health. (n.d.). Victoria State Government. https://www.betterhealth.vic.gov.au/health/healthyliving/exercise-and-mental-health

Fletcher, J. (2022, December 1). *What is the grey rock method and is it effective?* PsychCentral. https://psychcentral.com/health/grey-rock-method

Gupta, S. (2024, May 15). *How to identify and escape a narcissistic abuse cycle*. Verywell Mind. https://www.verywellmind.com/narcissistic-abuse-cycle-stages-impact-and-coping-6363187

Gupta, S. (2024, August 7). *Recognizing the signs of psychological abuse*. Verywell Mind. https://www.verywellmind.com/psychological-abuse-types-impact-and-coping-strategies-5323175

Heyl, J. C. (2023, December 19). *How to find a narcissistic abuse support group*. Verywell Mind.

https://www.verywellmind.com/how-to-find-a-narcissistic-abuse-support-group-5271477

Kaminski, H. (n.d.). *How to rebuild self-esteem after narcissistic abuse: Effective strategies for recovery.* Therapy Helpers. https://therapyhelpers.com/blog/rebuild-self-esteem-after-narcissistic-abuse/

Lachance, L., & Ramsey, D.(2015). Food, mood, and brain health: Implications for the modern clinician. *Mo Med, 112*(2), 11-15.

Lindner Center of HOPE. (2014, March 11). *Understanding narcissistic personality disorder.* Lindner Center of HOPE. https://lindnercenterofhope.org/blog/understanding-narcissistic-personality-disorder/

L.N. (2024, January 5). *The role of resilience in recovering from a narcissistic relationship.* Medium. https://medium.com/moving-forward-with-hope/the-role-of-resilience-in-recovering-from-a-narcissistic-relationship-824b7eaad3ad

Mayo Clinic.(n.d.). *Narcissistic personality disorder.* Mayo Clinic. https://www.mayoclinic.org/diseases-conditions/narcissistic-personality-disorder/symptoms-causes/syc-20366662

Mayo Clinic Staff. (2022, November 22). *Forgiveness: Letting go of grudges and bitterness.* Mayo Clinic. https://www.mayoclinic.org/healthy-lifestyle/adult-health/in-depth/forgiveness/art-20047692#

McBridge, K. (2008, September 23). *Will I ever be good enough? Healing the daughters of narcissistic mothers.* Free Press.

Moore, M. (2022, September 8). *The importance of personal boundaries.* PsychCentral. https://psychcentral.com/relationships/the-importance-of-personal-boundaries

Mughal, A. (n.d.). *Understanding narcissistic personality disorder: Insights and strategies* [Online course]. Alison. https://alison.com/course/understanding-narcissistic-personality-disorder-insights-and-strategies

Narcissistic abuse recovery books. (n.d.). Goodreads. https://www.goodreads.com/shelf/show/narcissistic-abuse-recovery

Newport Institute. (n.d.). *Identifying gaslighting: Signs, examples, and seeking help.* Newport Institute. https://www.newportinstitute.com/resources/mental-health/what_is_gaslighting_abuse/

Reid, S. (n.d.). *Codependency.* HelpGuide.org. https://www.helpguide.org/relationships/social-connection/codependency

Sandhu, M. (2022, February 21). *The benefits of journaling for mental health & healing.* Freedom. https://www.freedomaddiction.ca/blog/benefits-of-journaling-for-mental-health/

Scott, E. (2023, September 26). *How to use assertive communication.* Verywell Mind. https://www.verywellmind.com/learn-assertive-communication-in-five-simple-steps-3144969

Shafir, H. (2024, November 25). *Stages of healing after narcissistic abuse.* Choosing Therapy.

https://www.choosingtherapy.com/stages-of-healing-after-narcissistic-abuse/

Short, P. (2024, October 9). *Domestic violence: Understanding, healing, and reclaiming power.* Michigan Technological University. https://blogs.mtu.edu/belonging/2024/10/09/domestic-violence-understanding-healing-and-reclaiming-power/

Stanborough, J. (2023, June 5). *How to change negative thinking with cognitive restructuring.* Healthline. https://www.healthline.com/health/cognitive-restructuring

Taylor Counseling Group. (2024, April 2). *The 7 most common narcissistic manipulation tactics – and how you can deal with them.* https://taylorcounselinggroup.com/blog/how-to-deal-with-narcissistic-manipulation-tactics/

Thompson, E. (n.d.). *What is the best therapy for narcissistic abuse? Discover effective healing techniques.* Therapy Helpers. https://therapyhelpers.com/blog/what-is-the-best-therapy-for-narcissistic-abuse/?srsltid=AfmBOop0O2-b--hBr_p3l4PvaikdS8_1TbKPYQ4eM2MT-2uj8yVnn8v0

Villines, Z. (2023, December 20). *What is gray rocking?* Medical News Today. https://www.medicalnewstoday.com/articles/grey-rock#what-is-it

Website Director. (n.d.). *Breaking the silence: Surviving narcissistic abuse by survivor Patti.* BTSADV.

https://breakthesilencedv.org/breaking-the-silence-surviving-narcissistic-abuse-by-patti-r/

Westover, T. (2018, February 20). *Educated*. Random House.

www.ingramcontent.com/pod-product-compliance
Lightning Source LLC
LaVergne TN
LVHW012021060526
838201LV00061B/4402